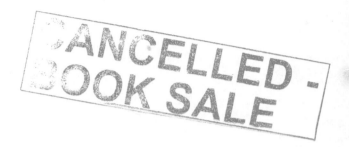
CONTRACEPTION
HEALTHY CHOICES

CONTRACEPTION
HEALTHY CHOICES
A CONTRACEPTIVE CLINIC IN A BOOK

2ND EDITION

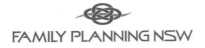

FAMILY PLANNING NSW

UNSW
PRESS

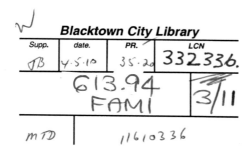
A UNSW Press book

Published by
University of New South Wales Press Ltd
University of New South Wales
Sydney NSW 2052
AUSTRALIA
www.unswpress.com.au

© FPA Health 2002, Family Planning NSW 2009
First edition published 2002
This edition 2009

National Library of Australia
Cataloguing-in-Publication entry
      Author: Family Planning NSW.
      Title: Contraception - healthy choices: a contraceptive clinic in a book /
      Family Planning NSW.
      Edition: 2nd ed.
      ISBN: 978 1 7422 3136 5 (pbk.)
      Subjects: Contraception.
        Contraceptives.
      Dewey Number: 363.96

Written and illustrated by Merri Collier
Medical consultant Dr Christine Read
Design Josephine Pajor-Markus
Cover Dreamstime
Printer Ligare

This book is printed on paper using fibre supplied from plantation or sustainably
managed forests.

CONTENTS

FOREWORD

Family Planning NSW has been informing women and their partners about contraception for more than 80 years. In 1926, when we first opened our doors, early changes to the roles of women in society were being felt in Australia. Women gained the vote in Australia before many other countries, and in South Australia were the first to be able to stand for parliament. The First World War had brought women into the workforce; women were attending university and becoming teachers, nurses and doctors in small but increasing numbers. These early changes to the long-held position of women as wives, mothers and nurturers were accompanied by a need for women to control their reproductive capacity. Until then, men had held the only key to preventing an unwanted pregnancy by using either withdrawal or the so-called 'prophylactic' (or condom). Contraception for women was championed by Dr Marie Stopes in England, and the first family planning clinic opened in London in 1921, as the 'Mother's Clinic'.

The diaphragm, introduced to Australia in the 1920s, was the first contraceptive method controlled by women. In those days, the diaphragm was only available to married women, and even then it was supplied in a rather secretive manner. It wasn't until almost 50 years ago that the era of the 'planned' and 'wanted' pregnancy, and the end of the 'unplanned' pregnancy, was thought to have finally arrived when the first oral contraceptive pills were launched in Australia and made widely available to women. In 1971, a major survey of fertility and family formation in Australia found that more than a third of non-pregnant fertile women were using the combined oral contraceptive pill. During the same decade, the use of the diaphragm fell from 21 per cent to 5 per cent and another important technological development arrived, the intrauterine device, which was used by 10 per cent of women in 1971.

During the 1970s, '80s and '90s, there were refinements of existing technologies such as the oral contraceptive pill, leading to the development of pills with lower doses of hormones, different dosage cycles or 'phases', and different types of the hormone progestogen. Society was once again changing; the need to prevent unwanted pregnancies was still important, but had come to be seen as 'normal', and what women wanted were safer and better contraceptives.

In the 2000s, there has been an emphasis on long-acting reversible methods of contraception (LARCs). With our increasingly busy lifestyles, methods that require daily use (such as the Pill) are often forgotten, and unplanned pregnancy has become all too common among women who are using contraception. A survey published in 2008 reported that more than 50 per cent of Australian women who had an unplanned pregnancy said they were using a contraceptive method at the time they became pregnant. The main reason for this is the inconsistent use of methods such as the Pill, diaphragms and condoms.

The first of the LARCs was the contraceptive implant, which sits just under the skin and provides contraceptive cover for three years. A second new method was the hormone containing IUD, which not only provides contraception but, true to the new desire for 'more than a contraceptive', has been used to treat women with heavy menstruation. The most recent technology to appear on the Australian scene has been the vaginal ring, which releases hormones similar to those in the Pill, and can be left in place for up to three weeks.

As technologies have developed, so too has our knowledge on how to use contraceptives. The World Health Organization and family planning organisations produce expert guidelines on safety and practice, and this area of medical knowledge has become specialised in its own right. Family Planning NSW is a member organisation of the national family planning body, Sexual Health and Family Planning Australia, and doctors can undertake specific training and gain a nationally recognised certificate in this discipline.

Fertility control is not, however, just a question of the availability of contraception. It must always be considered within its social context and tailored to individual circumstances. The contraceptive method that is appropriate for a woman at 20 years of age is likely to be different to that required at 40 years. Each woman and her partner needs to examine their particular requirements for contraception and discuss these with a clinician. This timely second edition of *Contraception – Healthy Choices* will be most helpful in guiding readers through all the options that are currently available.

Dr Christine Read
Medical Director, Family Planning NSW

INTRODUCTION

People tell us they want to make their own choices about the contraception they use. They want to know about each method and have time to think about which one they would prefer – one that suits their lifestyle now.

When you are choosing a method of contraception there are lots of things to consider. This book gives you clear information about the range of contraceptives available in Australia, and answers many questions that will help you choose one that is right for you. This is really important, because the reason most methods fail is because they are not used correctly, or sometimes because they are not used at all!

People are more likely to use something if they feel comfortable and confident about it. So take your time to read and think about which methods might suit you. The next step may be to go to your doctor or Family Planning centre to talk about it a bit more before you decide. It's also good to have a health check to make sure you can use the contraceptive method you choose. You will certainly need a check-up if you want to take the Pill or use another method that involves using hormones.

It is very important that you feel happy with the method you choose. If you are not happy about using it, your anxiety or discomfort could end up making you feel tense about sex, which could make you even unhappier. It could also affect your relationship with your sexual partner.

If you are anxious or uncomfortable about using a particular contraceptive method then it's worth asking yourself why you feel that way. Perhaps it is not acceptable in your culture for you to touch your vagina to insert a vaginal ring, or perhaps you don't like the idea of using something like the Pill because it affects your whole system. When you know the reason, you can decide whether you want to do something about it or just look for another method that you feel happier using.

You will need to find out whether you can get the method easily. For example, if you don't live in the city, you'll need to find a doctor in your area who is trained to insert intrauterine devices (IUDs) or implants. If you want to have a tubal ligation then it may be necessary to have time away from family or work commitments.

You also need to be able to afford the method you would like to use. For example, you may want to choose an IUD, but even though this works out to be a fairly inexpensive method over time, the cost can be quite high when you first pay for it.

Other things that may influence your choice are your age, and how you feel about the way a particular method may affect you or the possibility of you having children in the future. The method you choose could also depend on how effective you need it to be and whether an unexpected pregnancy would be a real problem to you at the moment.

You will probably find that you use different methods at different times in your life. There may be a time when you want a method that will be easy to keep private. Sometimes it could be worth using a method that protects you from sexually transmissible infections (STIs) as well, particularly if you have a new partner, or you have sex with more than one person, or your partner has sex with more than one person. If you are breastfeeding, you should consider using a method that would not have any effect on your milk supply.

If you use drugs or drink alcohol regularly, you may need to choose a method that you don't have to remember to use just before you have sex. If you have a physical disability, think about whether you have sufficient movement in your hands to use a particular method, for example, a female condom. You may need to have regular check-ups to make sure you can still use a method if you have a progressive disease. Your choice of contraception could also be affected if you have any loss of sexual sensation. Talk to your doctor to make sure the method you choose will not worsen any medical conditions you have. If you have an intellectual disability, make sure that you know all about the method and that you feel it is easy to use.

These are general things to think about. The sessions that follow will deal with more specific issues. If you are already having sex and you are not using contraception and you don't want to be pregnant, go to Chapter 2, which deals with male and female condoms. Condoms are a good method to start with, and you will be protecting yourself against unwanted pregnancy and sexually transmissible infections (STIs) while you are choosing the method that will suit you best.

ABOUT THE SESSIONS

As this is 'a contraceptive clinic in a book', each chapter presents information in the form of a clinic session. In each session, I give you information about a different method of contraception. I have imagined that you are a woman who has come to a clinic session and I speak directly to you. If you are a man reading this book, 'Hello, good to meet you too!' Oh yes, and when I talk about sexual intercourse or making love, I am going to call it 'having sex'.

In each session, I answer a set of questions about a particular contraceptive method. These are listed below. I've also added some questions you could ask yourself, to help you choose one that feels right for you. The questions I will answer in each session are:

What is (the method)?

When you find out, ask yourself 'Does that sound like something I might use?' If you answer 'Yes' or 'Maybe', find out more about it. If you answer 'No', you might want to look for one that sounds better to you.

Are there different types of (the method)?

Once you've read about the different types, ask yourself 'Which type would suit me best?'

How does it work?

When you know, ask yourself 'Do I feel confident that this method is worth using?' If you answer 'Yes', find out more about it. If you answer 'No' then keep looking.

How effective is it?

When doctors talk about the effectiveness of a method of contraception they usually mean 'How many women out of 100 will not become pregnant if they use that method for a year?' To make it simpler, I have referred to it as a percentage. The effectiveness is often recorded as a range, for example, we might say a method is 80 to 90 per cent effective. The higher number refers to the effectiveness if the method is always used exactly according to the instructions. The lower number might include human error.

Once you know how effective a method is, ask yourself 'Is that okay with me?' If the method is very effective, you will probably say 'Yes'. If it is not quite so effective, your answer will depend on how devastating it would be for you to become pregnant while you were using it. For example, if you intend to have a child in the next couple of years then you may not mind taking some risk if the method suits you in other ways. In this case, find out more to help you decide. Just remember that no method is 100 per cent effective. Well, abstinence is 100 per cent effective but that means you don't have sex at all.

In each session we discuss the question, Why would I want to choose the method? If you think the reasons we mention apply to you, then find out more.

We also look at the question, Are there any reasons why I could not use this method? If you find out that you cannot use a certain method, look further.

How do I use it?

Once you understand how to use a method, ask yourself 'Do I feel comfortable about using this method?' If your answer is 'Yes', carry on. If you feel concerned about anything, talk to a doctor or nurse or ring a Family Planning centre (the contact numbers are at the end of this book) to see if your worries can be cleared up.

Other questions that we will discuss are, Where do I get it? and What does it cost?

I will also answer some frequently asked questions about each method, and suggest some things you may want to think about if you are really considering a particular method. At the end of each session there is a short list of words from that session and how to pronounce them.

If you have any more questions or concerns as you learn about each method, write them down so you don't forget, and ask your local doctor or a doctor or nurse at a Family Planning centre. At the back of this book, there are contact details for Family Planning centres in each State, and suggestions about other places where you can get help on contraception issues.

1

BODIES, AND HOW PREGNANCY HAPPENS

A WOMAN'S BODY

Hello and welcome. We're going to begin by talking about bodies. I'll just take you through a quick refresher of the parts of men's and women's bodies that are involved in sex and reproduction. This will help you to understand how the different methods of contraception work.

Let's start with the woman's body. Look at the diagram that shows the parts we can see between a woman's legs (page 2). Right at the very front of the body there is pubic hair. Then, close to the front of her body you can see a spot on the diagram. This represents a little bump with a hood of skin over it. It is about the size of a pea, and it is called the clitoris. The clitoris is very sensitive. It plays a major part in the wonderful sensations that lead up to orgasm.

A bit behind the clitoris is a small opening to the urethra. The urethra is the passage that carries urine, or 'wee' as some people call it, from the bladder. Urine comes out of here when

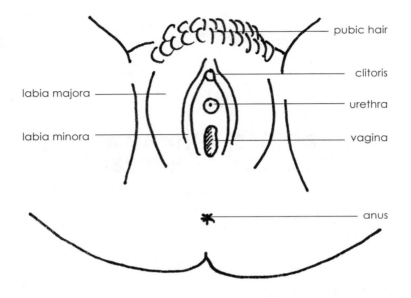

Female reproductive parts (external view)

we go to the toilet.

The next opening behind that is the vagina. It is a larger opening with a strong muscle around it, and it can also stretch a lot. You can insert a tampon here, and the muscle around the opening keeps the tampon inside. It stretches to allow a penis to enter during sex, and it can even stretch wide enough to allow a baby's head to pass through during childbirth.

Covering the clitoris and the openings to the urethra and the vagina are flaps of skin or vaginal lips. They are called labia. There are two labia majora, the outside ones, and two labia minora, the inside ones. The labia majora have quite thick skin and are covered with pubic hair. They protect the more delicate skin of the labia minora and the parts we have just talked about, which are called the genitals.

Closest to the back of the body is a third opening called the anus. Faeces, 'poo' or waste from the bowel comes out here when you go to the toilet.

Because we will be talking about how contraception works in your body, we'll look at the internal reproductive parts that you really need to know about. These are the vagina, the cervix, the uterus, the fallopian tubes and the ovaries.

Now look at the illustration on page 4. This diagram shows a woman's internal reproductive parts from the front. The vagina is a passage that leads to the uterus, or womb. It is usually between 6 and 10 centimetres long. When there is nothing inside it, the sides move together so that it looks like there is no space inside and it is closed. The vaginal walls are loose and have folds. They can stretch easily too.

At the far end of the vagina is the cervix. The cervix is actually the lower part of the uterus. It is made of thick pink muscle that feels a bit like the tip of your nose. You can feel it if you put your finger right up inside your vagina. If you want to feel for it, it's best to lean forward and have one foot up on a chair, or lie on your back with your knees bent up. You will need to slant your finger towards the small of your back to find it.

In the centre of the cervix is a very small opening called the os, which leads to the cervical canal that goes through to the space inside the uterus. During childbirth, the cervix gets thinner and opens up to allow the baby to pass through. Our bodies are amazing!

The uterus is shaped like an upside-down pear. It is normally about 6 centimetres long and 3 centimetres wide. It is made of very strong muscle that can not only stretch to accommodate a growing baby, but can also contract so strongly during childbirth that it pushes the baby out.

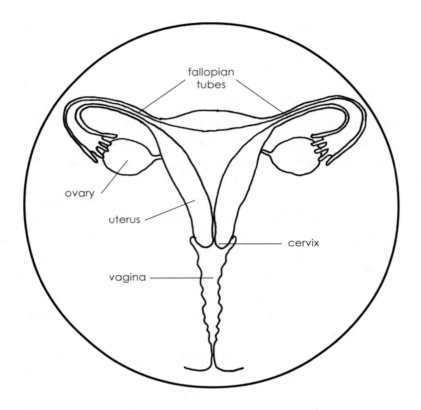

Female reproductive parts (front view)

The walls of the uterus are quite thick. On either side, close to the top, there is a fallopian tube. The fallopian tubes are long and very thin. They are hollow, and they join on to the uterus at one end and hover over the ovaries at the other. The ends closest to the ovaries flare out like trumpets, and have tiny finger-like structures called fimbria.

There is an ovary on each side of the uterus. They are joined to the uterus by strong bands of tissue that anchor them in place. Each ovary is about the size of an olive and contains

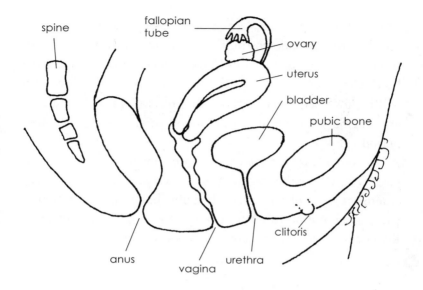

Female reproductive parts (side view)

thousands of tiny egg follicles with the potential to produce mature eggs. All these follicles were present when the woman was born.

Girls usually go through puberty sometime from about 11 to 15 years old. At puberty, hormonal changes occur in a girl's body so that the eggs, or ova, start to mature and the ovaries release them as they mature, at the rate of about one a month. This is called ovulation. Girls start having periods at this time. A woman usually continues to ovulate about once a month, unless she is pregnant or using hormonal contraception, until she is about 50 years old. During the years that she is ovulating, about 300 to 500 eggs are released.

At ovulation, the egg bursts out of the ovary and is funnelled into a fallopian tube, where it lives for about 24 hours as it travels down towards the uterus. If the woman has sex at this time and the egg meets a sperm and is fertilised, it takes about ten days to travel down the tube and implant in the lining of the uterus. If the egg does not meet a sperm and become fertilised within 24 hours, it will still travel down the tube and will be absorbed by the uterus, or will pass out of her uterus and vagina with the menstrual blood when she has her next period.

A woman's reproductive parts are shown from the side on page 5. See how the vagina tilts to the back. You can also see where the front of the pelvis, the pubic bone, sits in relation to the vagina and uterus. You may want to refer to this diagram if you choose a barrier method of contraception.

 HOW TO SAY THESE WORDS

anus *ay-niss*

cervix *ser-vicks*

clitoris *clit-or-iss*

contraception *con-tra-sep-shun*

embryo *em-bree-yo*

faeces *fee-sees*

fallopian *fal-owe-pee-yan*

fimbria *fim-bree-ya*

genitals *gen-it-als*

labia *lay-bee-ya*

menopause *men-owe-paws*

orgasm *or-gaz-im*

ovaries *owe-ver-ees*

ovulation *ov-you-lay-shun*

puberty *pew-ber-tee*

pubic *pew-bick*

urethra *you-reeth-ra*

uterus *you-ter-iss*

vagina *va-gine-a*

A MAN'S BODY

Now we'll go on to the man's reproductive parts. Look at the illustration opposite. This shows you what you can see on the outside of a man's body between his legs. In this case, imagine he is leaning back rather than lying flat. At the front of

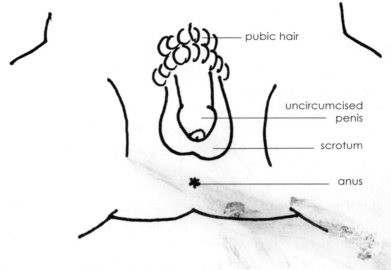

Male reproductive parts (external view)

his body you can see pubic hair, and under that is his penis. Penises come in a range of sizes, and can look quite small when they are in their normal state. By 'normal' I mean when they are not aroused, but are soft and hanging loosely. They have a shaft that is several centimetres long, which starts at the lowest part of a man's abdomen and ends with a sort of bulb-shaped part that is called the glans. The glans has a different type of skin to the shaft, it is more sensitive, and at the tip of the glans is a little opening to the urethra. Urine, or wee, comes out of here when a man goes to the toilet.

When a baby boy is born he has a fold of skin covering the glans. This is called the foreskin. It is open at the end, just beyond the tip of the glans, so that the opening to the urethra is not covered. The foreskin can be pulled back when the penis is washed, and it moves back to expose the more sensitive skin of the glans when the man has sex. A penis that has a foreskin is said to be uncircumcised.

Some men have been circumcised. That means that the foreskin has been removed. Usually this is done by a doctor, or by a religious elder, when the baby is very young. In some cultures it is done at puberty. Occasionally a man may need to be circumcised later in life for medical reasons.

When a man becomes sexually excited, or 'turned on', his penis becomes erect, which means it gets harder and larger. When a man has an erection, it is difficult to tell if he has been circumcised or not because the foreskin pulls back to expose the glans. The penis gets harder and larger because blood flows to spongy tissue in the penis and fills it. The passage from the bladder that carries urine is blocked off so that when he ejaculates, or comes, only semen, which is the fluid containing sperm, is released.

Directly behind the penis is a loose bag of skin called the scrotum. Inside the scrotum are the two testes, or balls, that produce sperm. Sometimes the scrotum hangs loosely, and sometimes it scrunches up tightly close to the body. This generally depends on how the man is built. It can also happen because sperm need to be kept at a certain temperature to live, and so when it is hot, the testes may be kept cooler by hanging more loosely away from the body, and when it is cold, they can move up close to keep warmer.

Behind the scrotum, towards the back of the body, is an opening, which is the man's anus. Faeces, or waste from the bowel, comes out here when the man goes to the toilet.

Now let's look inside the man's body (page 9). This shows the man's body from the side. Perhaps it would be best to start with sperm production. Look at the testes inside the scrotum. They are about the size of walnuts and are made up of tightly coiled tubes where sperm and hormones are pro-

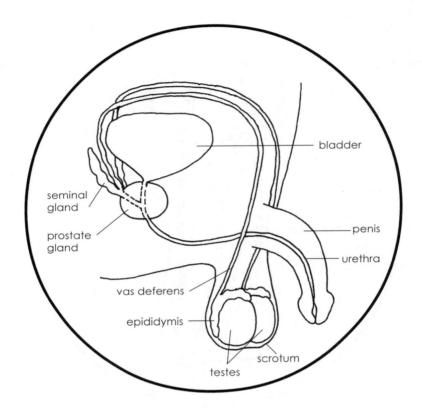

Male reproductive parts (side view)

duced from puberty onward. Sperm are really tiny and you can only see them if you use a microscope. You may have heard of testosterone. This is one of the hormones produced in the testes. It is involved in producing male characteristics such as body hair and a deep voice.

Along the back to the top of each testis is the epididymis. The epididymis stores more mature sperm waiting to be fed into the vas deferens when they are needed. The vas deferens is usually just called the 'vas'. One vas leads away from each

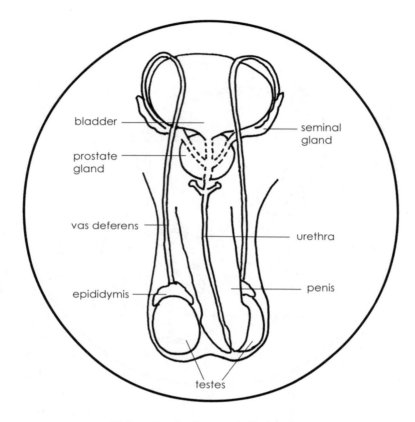

bladder

prostate
gland

vas deferens

epididymis

seminal
gland

urethra

penis

testes

Male reproductive parts (front view)

testis. They are long and narrow and carry sperm to the urethra. The vas loop around the bladder and as they feed into
the prostate gland the sperm mix with semen, which is fluid
from the seminal glands. The prostate is also where the part of
the urethra that is connected to the bladder can be closed off,
so that only semen is released when a man ejaculates.

Now that you know what all the parts are, look at the illustration above. This shows inside the man's body from the
front. It does look rather complicated, but if you look carefully,

and refer to the diagram of the side view, you can work out where all the parts fit.

HOW TO SAY THESE WORDS

circumcised *sir-cum-sized*   prostate *pross-tate*

ejaculate *ee-jack-you-late*   scrotum *skroe-tim*

epididymis *eppy-diddy-mis*   testosterone *tess-toss-ter-own*

erection *a-reck-shun*   vas deferens *vass deff-are-enz*

penis *pee-niss*

HOW DOES A PREGNANCY START?

So how does a pregnancy start? Well, pregnancy starts with sex between a man and a woman. When people are having sex, after some time, when the man is sexually aroused and hopefully the woman is too, he puts his penis into her vagina and as he moves backwards and forwards, her vagina becomes more engorged and sensitive. Those feelings build up and up until he, or they, experience orgasm, when the muscles around the genital area contract strongly again and again and a sensation of intense pleasure and then relaxation follows.

I'll explain that again, focussing on the mechanics. Basically, when the man is aroused his penis becomes hard. During sexual activity, he puts his penis into the woman's vagina. With further stimulation, he has an orgasm and ejaculates, which means that semen, containing sperm, spurts out from his penis.

When the man ejaculates inside the vagina, tens of millions of sperm rush up through the cervix into the uterus. Many find their way into the fallopian tubes. Most get lost and die on the way, but if there is a newly released egg in one of the fallopian tubes, the first sperm to reach the egg and burrow through its protective coating will start a new pregnancy. This is called fertilisation and when a sperm fertilises an egg, we call that conception. Once the egg is fertilised, no other sperm can penetrate it, and it travels down the fallopian tube and implants in the lining of the uterus, where it starts to grow.

In the following sessions you will learn all about the different ways to prevent conception. This is called contraception.

 HOW TO SAY THESE WORDS

conception *con-sep-shun*
contraception *con-tra-sep-shun*
fertilisation *fer-till-eye-zay-shun*

2

BARRIER METHODS OF CONTRACEPTION

THE MALE CONDOM

Well, this is our first session about the different methods of contraception and you've told me you'd like to find out all you can about condoms. When I talk about condoms in this session, I will mean male condoms. There is a female condom that fits inside a woman's vagina rather than on a man's penis, but we'll talk about that in the next session.

What is a condom?

A condom is a thin covering that a man wears on his penis when the penis is erect, that is, when it is hard or stiff. The man wears it when he is having sex to prevent pregnancy. Most condoms are made of latex rubber, but non-latex condoms that are made from a type of plastic are also available. Condoms are shaped like a tube that is closed at one end (page 14), and they fit very closely over the penis like a second skin.

Generally condoms are a light creamy brown colour, with a thin rim at the open end, and the closed end is either plain and rounded, or has a little teat- or nipple-shaped space right at the tip.

Are there different types of condoms?

You can also get lots of different types of condoms. They come in a range of colours, including red, blue and black. You can choose special flavours such as strawberry and banana. There are several different shapes. You can get straight, flared or contoured and some have ribbed or dotted textures. Condoms can have different-shaped ends, and you can get them already lubricated, or lubricated with spermicide.

Fancy condoms are not always as reliable as the plain ones and it is a good idea to read the label on the packet to be sure they are meant to be used for protection against pregnancy and sexually transmissible infections (STIs), and not just as novelty items.

Some condoms are made of stronger, thicker latex than others, and some are made of very fine latex. Generally they

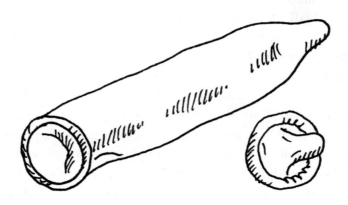

Condoms

are one size fits all. This is because although penises are different sizes when they are soft, they all tend to be about the same size when they are erect. You can get condoms that are a tighter fit, and condoms that are contoured may suit men who want them slightly smaller. Condoms that are flared sometimes suit men who want them slightly larger.

How do condoms work?

A condom forms a barrier that stops sperm getting into the woman's body. That is why it is called a barrier method of contraception. When a man ejaculates or comes, the semen (that is, the fluid that contains sperm) comes out of the penis into the tip of the condom and collects there. Because it doesn't go into the woman's body, the sperm cannot join with an egg to start a pregnancy. There is also much less chance of passing on a sexually transmissible infection (STI).

How effective are condoms?

Condoms are about 90 per cent effective. This means that if the partners of 100 women used condoms as their method of contraception for a year, about 10 of those women would become pregnant. People sometimes say they use condoms as their method of contraception, but what they don't say is that they do not use a condom every time they have sex. The effectiveness rate is higher for condoms if you actually use one every time you have sex, and you put it on before you have any penis-in-vagina sex. It is also higher if you use condoms correctly every time, taking care when you put it on and take it off and using a water-based lubricant with latex condoms, because this reduces the risk of the condom breaking. You should only use each condom once and then throw it away, otherwise there's a much greater risk of pregnancy.

Why would I want to choose condoms?

Condoms not only reduce the risk of pregnancy; they are the only method of contraception that can also protect you against sexually transmissible infections (STIs), including HIV/AIDS. You may want to use condoms if you have a new sexual partner, or more than one sexual partner, or if your partner has sex with other people. Condoms may be a good choice if you don't have sex regularly so you don't want to use something that affects your body all the time.

There is no legal age limit for using condoms. And there is no need to see a doctor to get them. They are not expensive and there are no serious medical side effects to using condoms.

Are there any reasons why I could not use condoms?

There may be reasons why you don't want to use condoms. A small number of people may be allergic to latex rubber or a particular lubricant. However, this is very rare. Non-latex condoms can be a good alternative for people who are allergic to latex. If you or your sexual partner gets a rash or has any discomfort around your genitals, that is, your penis or vagina, check with your doctor or clinic.

Where do I get condoms?

You can buy condoms and water-based lubricant at Family Planning centres, chemists, Sexual Health clinics, vending machines, supermarkets, petrol stations, and by mail order.

What do condoms cost?

You can buy latex condoms in their own little packets, one at a time, for about 25 cents at Family Planning centres. The average cost is about $7 to $12 for packs of 12, from supermarkets, chemists and online. Non-latex condoms cost about $22 to

HOW DO I USE A CONDOM?

Each condom comes in its own little packet.

To put on the condom

1   The first thing you do is tear open the packet, taking care not to tear the condom with your fingernails or the sharp edge of a ring while you are opening the packet or taking the condom out. You can push the condom out of the way while it is still inside the packet before you start.

2   The condom will be rolled up and will look like a circle of loose fine rubber with a thick rim. The rim is actually the body of the condom tightly rolled up. As you hold it while it is still rolled up, check that the rim is rolled towards the centre on the side facing you. This is important, so that when you unroll the condom over the penis, it will roll down easily.

3   Hold the edge of the rolled-up condom with one hand. With the thumb and first finger of your other hand, take hold of the loose part at the centre of the circle and squeeze it. This ensures there is space at the end of the condom to collect the semen when the man comes. Some condoms have a special little shape like a teat or nipple, at their closed end, especially for this.

4   The penis must be erect before you put the condom on it.

5   While the condom is still rolled up, and you are still holding the tip squeezed between your thumb and first finger, put the condom on the head of the penis like a cap.

6   Using the thumb and first two fingers of your other hand, roll the condom all the way down so that it covers the penis, with the rim of the condom around the base of the penis. Make sure there is still space at the tip to collect the semen.

7   Put some water-based lubricant on the condom.

8   Now you can safely have sex.

To remove

1   After sex and before the penis has become soft, you need to hold onto the condom at the base of the penis so that the condom does not come off and semen does not leak out, and carefully pull away from your partner.

2   Point the penis down, hold the condom just behind the teat to keep the semen in and pull the condom off.

3   Tie a knot in the open end of the condom to keep the semen inside.

4   Wrap the condom in a tissue, paper towel or plastic bag, and put it in the bin. Do not flush it down the toilet because condoms do not dissolve, and the toilet could get blocked.

$30 for packs of 10. Water-based lubricant comes in single-use packets that cost about 25 cents at Family Planning centres, and in tubes for between $4 and $10.

Frequently asked questions about condoms

Q Why do condoms break?

A Latex rubber is perishable, which means that it can harden and crack or tear easily after a certain period of time. Heat and humidity can also affect latex rubber, so condoms should be kept in a cool, dry place.

It is best to buy condoms from somewhere that is air-conditioned like a supermarket, and not where they have been stored in the sun. Do not keep condoms in the glove box of your car. If you keep them in your wallet, throw them out after a week.

Condoms should be used before the expiry date on the packet; otherwise, the latex may have perished and they are very likely to break. You should not use oil-based lubricants like petroleum jelly or massage oil with latex condoms, because these can make the condoms break too.

Condoms may break because you have not used enough water-based lubricant. They can also break if you don't leave enough space at the end of the condom for the semen to collect.

Q Why do condoms slip off?

A Condoms may slip off if you wait too long after ejaculation before withdrawing because the penis gets softer and smaller in size.

Q Why do condoms sometimes leak even though they are not broken?

A Condoms may leak from the open edge if you wait too long after ejaculation before withdrawing because the penis gets softer and smaller and the condom doesn't fit tightly any more. They may also leak if you don't roll them down far enough on the penis.

Things to think about if you are considering condoms

» It is important to feel comfortable with your method of contraception, because if you don't, you are less likely to use it every time you have sex. And sex is meant to feel good too, so it's better not to be tense about your contraception. On the other hand, if you don't want to be pregnant then you need to use something, and all methods have their good and bad points. If condoms seem the best choice for you but you feel a bit uncomfortable about using them, it is worth making an effort for a while, because condoms have the advantage of protecting against sexually transmissible infections (STIs) as well.

» While some people think that condoms are messy or that putting them on interrupts the natural flow of sex, other people have made putting on the condom a natural and sensuous part of having sex and they really like it.

» Some men say that wearing a condom makes their penis less sensitive, so they don't enjoy sex as much as they do without a condom. Sometimes this is because the condom is too tight over the head of the penis. It is worth trying a different type of condom, for example, one that is flared may feel better because its shape allows a bit more room for the head of the penis.

» You will need to remember to have a supply of condoms and lubricant ready in case you need them.

» If a condom breaks when you have sex, it helps to have thought about what you would do. You can get emergency contraception from a chemist, but remember that a woman needs to take it within 120 hours (five days) of having unprotected sex for it to be effective.

HOW TO SAY THESE WORDS

 condom   *con-dom*

latex   *lay-tex*

lubricated   *loob-rick-ate-ed*

spermicide   *sperm-a-side*

THE FEMALE CONDOM

Now that we've talked about the male condom, I'll tell you about the female condom!

What is a female condom?

A female condom looks like a large, loose male condom but it has two big flexible rings, one at the closed end and one around the open end. It is about 17 centimetres long, and is wider than the male condom. It is made of polyurethane, which is a soft clear plastic, whereas you may remember that most male condoms are made of latex rubber. Each female condom comes already lubricated with a silicone-based lubricant.

You wear the female condom inside your vagina like a second skin. You use the ring at the closed end to help you slide

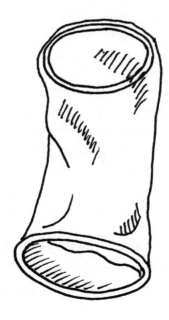

Female condom

the female condom into your vagina. The ring at the open end fits flat against your vulva, which is the area around your vagina. It is possible to remove the inner ring and use the female condom like a baggy male condom.

Are there different types of female condoms?

Right now, there is only one type of female condom available in Australia and it is called 'the female condom', which isn't hard to remember. It comes in only one size and it can fit anyone.

How do female condoms work?

Because the female condom forms a barrier that is like a second skin inside the vagina, when the man comes, the semen that has sperm in it stays inside the female condom. Sperm cannot get to the opening in the cervix and up into the fallopian tubes to meet an egg, so you don't get pregnant.

How effective are they?

The female condom is rated about 88 to 98 per cent effective. This means that if 100 women used the female condom as their method of contraception for one year, between 2 and 12 of them would have an unplanned pregnancy. You can see that if you use the female condom absolutely correctly every single time you have sex, it can be 98 per cent effective – so if you are committed to using it, it is very effective.

Why would I want to choose female condoms?

You may want to choose female condoms because, like male condoms, they not only help to protect you against pregnancy, but they also help to protect you against sexually transmissible infections (STIs).

Other reasons for choosing female condoms might be that you have tried male condoms and had a scare with one tearing, or if you or your partner are allergic to latex. Female condoms are stronger and less likely to tear than male condoms, and the polyurethane they are made from is unlikely to cause an allergic reaction. Because polyurethane conducts heat, some people say sex feels more natural than with latex male condoms. Polyurethane is also less likely to deteriorate in heat and light than latex.

Perhaps you think that condoms would suit your needs at the moment but, as a woman, you would prefer to have control over your own contraception. Using female condoms gives you that control. You can make sure you have them available and that you use them correctly every time you have sex.

You may want to choose female condoms because you only use them when you have sex, so your whole body is not affected. Another reason could be that you don't need to see a doctor before you can get them. If you want to, you can insert a female condom before you have sex so you don't have to be interrupted, and you don't have to be careful to remove it as soon as the man ejaculates or 'comes', the way you do with the male condom. You don't need to use spermicide for extra protection, and you can use a female condom when you have your periods.

Men tend to like the female condom because it doesn't feel tight around the penis like ordinary condoms do, and the penis doesn't have to be erect or hard before you can use the female condom.

Are there any reasons why I could not use the female condom?

There are no physical or medical reasons that would stop you from using the female condom.

HOW DO I USE THE FEMALE CONDOM?

The female condom comes in a packet that is small enough to fit in a handbag.

To insert

1   Carefully tear open the packet. Although the polyurethane that the female condom is made from is pretty strong, it is still possible to tear it with your fingernails or the sharp edge of a ring.

2   Rub the sides of the female condom together to spread around the lubricant that is already on it.

3   Look at the flexible ring around the open end. We'll call this the outer ring. There is another one at the closed end, and we'll call this the inner ring. If you know what a diaphragm looks like, the ring is about the same size as the rim of a diaphragm, and you put the inner ring into your vagina as though you were putting in a diaphragm.

4   Hold the inner ring between the thumb and middle finger of one hand.

5   Squeeze the inner ring to make a long thin shape.

6   With your other hand, hold the lips of your vagina apart.

7   Slide the female condom, while it is still squeezed, into your vagina and push it gently down and back as far as it will go. When it is in the right position you won't be able to feel it. Don't worry, it can't go too far inside you, and it won't hurt.

8   The outer ring should fit just outside the vagina.

9   Make sure the female condom is not twisted inside your vagina.

10 Just before you are going to have sex you may want to add more lubricant.

11 Guide the penis into the outer ring so that it doesn't go in between the female condom and your vaginal wall, or you could get pregnant.

After sex you don't have to remove the female condom right away, but it is best to take it out before you stand up.

To remove

1 Take hold of the outer ring, squeeze it and then twist it to keep the semen inside.
2 Pull the female condom out gently, wrap it in a plastic bag and throw it in the bin. Do not flush it down the toilet.
3 Each time you have sex use a new female condom.

Where do I get female condoms?

You can buy female condoms at Family Planning centres, Sexual Health clinics, some chemists, and online. Look in the back of this book for contact details.

What do they cost?

Female condoms cost about $2.90 each or $8 for a pack of three.

Frequently asked questions about female condoms

Q Can you use a female condom and a male condom at the same time to make extra sure you don't get pregnant?

A No, you should not use female condoms and male condoms together because the friction is likely to make them tear, and at least one or both of them could move out of place.

Q Can you use extra lubricant like baby oil or Vaseline with female condoms?

A Yes, it is actually good to use extra lubricant and because the female condom is made of a type of plastic, and not latex like the male condom, it is fine to use oil-based lubricant if you want to.

Q When I have sex the female condom keeps bunching up and getting pushed inside my vagina. What can I do?

A If that happens, put in more lubricant.

Things to think about if you are considering the female condom

» If you have a vaginal or pelvic infection you should get it treated before you use a female condom.

» Some people think that inserting a female condom inter-rupts sex and they don't want to do that, but you can put the female condom in place long before you start having sex if you want to.

» You will need to feel comfortable about touching your genitals.

» You can use each female condom only once and then you have to throw it away.

» Female condoms are more expensive than male condoms.

» It takes a little while to get comfortable inserting the female condom. It may take a few attempts to get it in the right position, but it is very easy to insert once you get used to it.

» It can also take a little while to get used to the feel and sometimes the sound it makes during sex, which can be like a rustling noise, but after a while you probably won't notice it at all.

» Not all chemists stock the female condom. If you cannot buy them from a store near you, you may need to plan ahead and order a supply online.

HOW TO SAY THESE WORDS
polyurethane *polly-you-ree-thain*

DIAPHRAGMS

Now we'll talk about diaphragms. You might have heard about diaphragms and caps. They are quite similar in the way they work, but we'll just talk about diaphragms now and discuss cervical caps next.

What is a diaphragm?

A diaphragm looks like a little round shallow bowl, on average about 6–8 centimetres across and 2 centimetres deep. It is usually made of soft latex rubber that is a creamy colour. You wear it inside your vagina. It covers the cervix and the upper part of your vagina. It has a rim that is firm but flexible and can be squeezed into a narrow oval shape so that you can slide it into your vagina easily.

Diaphragms are made in a range of sizes. It is not safe to go and buy one the same size as your friend's just because you wear the same size in clothes. You will need a doctor or nurse to examine you and tell you what size is right for you. It has to do with the length of the vagina and the position of the cervix and pubic bone, and the size you need can change if you change weight or have a baby.

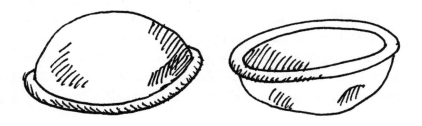

Diaphragm

Are there different types of diaphragms?

The type of diaphragm that is available in Australia at present is the arcing-spring or All-flex diaphragm.

The All-flex diaphragm has a strong and flexible spring inside the latex rim, which holds the diaphragm firmly in place by pressing against the walls of your vagina. This sounds like it could be uncomfortable, but if the diaphragm is the right size for you and it is in the correct position, you can't feel it. The rim of this diaphragm bends into a 'C' shape, which can make it easier to put in place behind the cervix.

The doctor or nurse who fits you with a diaphragm will decide which size you need. Basically it will be the one that fits best in your vagina so that it presses firmly against the vaginal walls without slipping out of place.

How does a diaphragm work?

The diaphragm forms a barrier across the cervix so that most sperm cannot get up into the uterus and tubes to meet an egg. If a sperm doesn't join with an egg then you cannot get pregnant.

You may want to use spermicide with a diaphragm. We will talk about spermicide in a later session, but it is a special type of cream or gel. The idea is that if any sperms get around the edge of the diaphragm, the spermicide will kill them. It can be difficult to get spermicide in Australia at present, so if you want to use it and you cannot get it at a chemist, you may need to order it online. Tests have been done to see if diaphragms work better with spermicide. Results seem to show that diaphragms work almost as well without spermicide.

How effective are diaphragms?

If diaphragms are used correctly, they are 84 to 94 per cent effective. This means that if 100 women used diaphragms as their method of contraception for a year, between six and sixteen of them would have an unplanned pregnancy. Some people say they use a diaphragm as their method of contraception, but in fact they don't use it every time they have sex. Sometimes they forget to use it, or they haven't got it with them, or sometimes they just don't want to use it. If you don't use it all the time, it obviously can't work as well as it should.

Another reason for accidental pregnancies while using a diaphragm could be that the diaphragm was not covering the cervix. It can sometimes squeeze into the vagina in front of the cervix although it usually feels uncomfortable there, so you'd normally be aware that something wasn't right. Also, if you lose a lot of weight the diaphragm may not fit properly any more, and some sperm may be able to get around the rim and up through the cervix. These are good reasons to check that your diaphragm fits properly and is in the correct place.

Why would I want to choose a diaphragm?

You may want to use a diaphragm because you can insert it beforehand rather than during sex. Also, you only need to wear it when you have sex, so it does not affect your body all the time. Another good thing about the diaphragm is that it usually lasts for about two years. You just wash it and use it over and over again.

You can use a diaphragm when you are menstruating, that is, when you are having your periods. It can collect the blood for several hours, as long as your period isn't very heavy. It is particularly important that it is not left in place much longer than that when you have a period, because of the increased risk of infection.

Are there any reasons why I could not use a diaphragm?

You may not be able to use a diaphragm if your vagina can't hold the diaphragm properly in place, but you won't know that until you are examined.

You may not be able to use a latex diaphragm if you or your partner are allergic to latex rubber. The symptoms of an allergy like this are itching and soreness. It's best to go and have a check-up to make sure there is no other reason for the irritation. It could also be an infection. If you are using spermicide then that may be the cause, rather than the latex.

HOW DO I USE A DIAPHRAGM?

To insert

1 Wash your hands before taking the diaphragm out of its case.
2 Stand with one foot on a chair or the toilet or bath, or crouch down, or lie on your back with your knees bent up. Whatever position you prefer, you will need to be able to bend forward to feel that the diaphragm is in place.
3 Hold it with the rim of the diaphragm facing you so that, as you look at it, it looks like a little cup.
4 Hold the diaphragm in one hand with your thumb on one side of the rim and your first and second fingers on the other side of the rim. If you are normally right-handed then it is probably best to use your right hand. If you are left handed, use your left hand.
5 Squeeze your thumb and fingers together so that the diaphragm forms a narrow oval shape instead of a circle.
6 With your other hand, open your labia, which are the lips covering your vagina, and hold them apart.
7 You may want to check for the position of your vagina with a finger, if you are not used to touching yourself there.
8 Bend forward, and gently but firmly push the squeezed dia-

phragm into your vagina, tilting it down on an angle towards the small of your back. You may feel it slide into place as you find the correct angle.

9 The leading rim of the diaphragm should slip under the cervix and then come up against the vaginal wall.

10 Let the diaphragm go as it slips into place.

11 Slide your middle finger into your vagina and feel the rim of the diaphragm that is closest to the opening to your vagina.

12 Push the rim up until you feel it settle into place behind your pubic bone.

13 Using the same finger, feel the soft dome of the diaphragm to check that it is covering your cervix. You should feel a lump something like the end of your nose under the latex. If the latex just gives way easily and it feels flat underneath, the cervix isn't covered and the diaphragm has gone in front of it, along the wall of your vagina. Take the diaphragm out and start again.

To remove

1 Slide a finger into your vagina and firmly push it between the rim of the diaphragm and the wall of your vagina.

2 Hook your finger over the rim and pull the diaphragm forward and down. If you can remember to relax by breathing out, or even bearing down, as you do when you have a bowel movement, the diaphragm will slip out quite easily.

After you have had sex, you should leave the diaphragm in place for at least six hours because the sperm can live in your vagina for a while and it takes about six hours before you are safe from getting pregnant.

It is fine to leave your diaphragm in longer (overnight or even all day) but it's important to take it out and clean it within 24 hours or it may start to smell rather unpleasant. If you leave it in place for longer than that, there is also a slight risk you could get an infection. When you are not having periods, you can wear it all the time if you want to, apart from taking it out and washing it every 24 hours.

Occasionally, a diaphragm is difficult to remove. Don't worry because there is no way it can get lost inside you; it can't go past the end of your vagina. Take a couple of deep breaths and remind yourself that you *will* be able to get it out, and then try again. There's no rush. As a last resort you can always go to a clinic and get the doctor or nurse to take it out for you. And just because it is difficult to remove once does not mean it will be difficult again.

When you take it out, wash the diaphragm with soap and water and dry it thoroughly. You can dust it lightly with corn-flour so that it is completely dry, but don't use talcum powder, which has perfumes and preservatives. Keep it in its plastic container away from heat and light.

Where do I get them?

You need to go to a doctor to be fitted for a diaphragm. The doctor will tell you what size you need and show you how to use it. At Family Planning centres you can see a doctor and buy the diaphragm there. If you see your local doctor, you will then go and buy your diaphragm from a chemist. Many chemists don't keep diaphragms in stock, but will order them for you.

What does a diaphragm cost?

Diaphragms cost between $75 and $90.

What happens when I have a diaphragm fitted?

The practitioner who is fitting the diaphragm will often suggest that you make two appointments. One is to find out what size you need and how to use it, and the other is to check that you are using the diaphragm properly and that you are happy with it.

You can have a fitting for a diaphragm at any time, as long as you are not pregnant. If you have just had a baby, then you must wait at least six weeks from giving birth. It is also probably best to wait a couple of days if you have a heavy period.

The doctor or nurse fitting you will give you an internal examination. From this, they can work out approximately the right size for you. They might then try a couple of sizes in your vagina to make sure of the exact size. They will show you how to use the diaphragm and will usually give you one to take home and practise with for a week or so. While you are practising with it, you should use another method of contraception if you have sex. You might want to use condoms or the Pill or an intrauterine device (IUD) if you already have them.

On your second visit, the doctor or nurse will check to make sure you can use the diaphragm properly and that it is a good fit. If you decide that you want to keep using a diaphragm, you will then go and buy your own.

Some doctors will use special fitting rings to decide what size you need and then give you a prescription to pick up the right size from the chemist. You should have the size and fit of your diaphragm checked each time you have a Pap test. If you gain or lose four or five kilograms, or you have been pregnant, it's important to have an extra check-up in case you need a different size.

Frequently asked questions about diaphragms

Q Can I use a diaphragm if I am using a vaginal cream for thrush?

A You should not use latex diaphragms, caps or latex condoms if you are using vaginal creams for thrush because those creams are oil-based and they can damage latex. The latex could tear or crack or get a hole in it and then you could get pregnant. It is best to avoid penis-in-vagina sex until a week after you have finished the treatment for thrush.

Q Can a man feel the diaphragm when it's in place?

A Most men can't feel it and those who can don't usually think it's a problem. If your partner says it's uncomfortable, it may not be in the correct position.

Things to think about if you are considering using a diaphragm

» Women who use diaphragms have a greater risk of getting cystitis or bladder irritation than women who use other methods of contraception. One reason for this may be that the rim of the diaphragm is pressing on the outlet tube from the bladder. The diaphragm can also hold secretions and bacteria in the vagina for longer than usual and this can be the cause of infection.

» Some women don't like having to touch their genitals, that is, their labia and vagina, to insert a diaphragm, and for some women it is not culturally acceptable. If you are not comfortable about touching your genitals then the diaphragm may not be the right choice for you. It is important that you feel comfortable so that you can insert it properly without feeling so concerned that it stops you from enjoying sex.

» If the diaphragm moves out of place while you are having sex, or if after sex you find that it has a little tear or a hole in it, you may want to use emergency contraception. If you think you would want to use emergency contraception if this happened to you, find out where you can get it now so that you will know where to go if you need to. Read the section on emergency contraception for more information. You must take emergency contraception within 120 hours (five days) of having unprotected sex for it to work.

» It's important to have your diaphragm with you when you're going to have sex. You will need to remember to pack it if you go on holidays. You will need to carry it with you, or insert it beforehand, if you think there's any chance you might have sex when you're not at home.

» Some people think that having to insert a diaphragm interrupts sex, but you can put it in before you are going to have sex.

» Other people make inserting their diaphragm a natural and sensuous part of having sex.

» If you absolutely do not want a pregnancy at this time, then the diaphragm is probably not the right choice for you now.

» If you feel, after taking everything into account, that a diaphragm is the only choice for you, think seriously about what you would want to do if you got pregnant, so that you are prepared in case it happens.

» Oil-based products should not be used with diaphragms because they may damage the latex rubber. Products that are oil-based include baby oil, hand cream, petroleum jelly or Vaseline, massage oil and any anti-fungal creams or pessaries that you may be prescribed if you have thrush. Some spermicides are oil-based, so you should read the label to check.

HOW TO SAY THESE WORDS
cervical *ser-vick-ill*
cystitis *sis-tie-tis*
diaphragm *die-a-fram*

CERVICAL CAPS

What is a cervical cap?

Cervical caps are no longer available in Australia, but I will tell you about them in case you have heard about them or you decide to get one if you travel overseas. Cervical caps are similar to diaphragms but they are much smaller (page 36). A cervical cap just fits over the cervix like a little cap. Most people just call the cervical cap 'the Cap'.

Are there different types of cervical caps?

There are various types of caps available in other countries. They are usually made of latex rubber and are shaped like little bowls or thimbles or a combination of the two, and they all stick to the cervix, or to the cervix and the far end of the vagina, by suction.

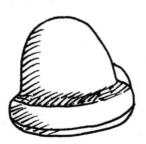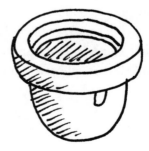

Cervical cap

How do cervical caps work?

Caps, like diaphragms, are barriers to sperm. The cap covers the cervix so that sperm cannot get into the uterus and tubes to meet an egg and start a pregnancy.

Some women use spermicide with a cap. We will talk about spermicide later. Tests have been done to see if caps work better with spermicide, but they seem to work almost as well without it.

How effective are cervical caps?

Cervical caps are between 82 to 90 per cent effective. If you use the cap correctly every time, it is much more reliable.

Why would I want to choose a cervical cap?

A cap may be a good choice for women who have tried a diaphragm but it didn't suit them. Some vaginal muscles aren't able to keep a diaphragm in place. If a diaphragm irritates your bladder, a cap could be a better option. Women who are inclined to put on weight and take it off fairly regularly could find that a cap is good because the size you need doesn't change with your weight.

Are there any reasons why I could not use a cervical cap?

Some women have the type of cervix that does not suit a cap. You won't know about this until you have been examined. You would not be able to use a cap if you or your partner are allergic to latex, but this is very rare.

HOW DO I USE A CERVICAL CAP?

Inserting a cap is quite similar to inserting a diaphragm. You will be shown how to use it if you are somewhere that has them available.

Where do I get cervical caps?

You cannot get cervical caps in Australia. You can only get them in some other countries. You would need to go to a doctor or nurse to find out what type of cap you need and the correct size for you, and to learn how to use it.

Frequently asked questions about cervical caps.

Q Are they as effective as the diaphragm?

A Cervical caps are about as effective as diaphragms.

Things to think about if you are considering using a cervical cap

Most of the issues are the same as for the diaphragm, but there are a few differences.

» A cervical cap is not as likely as a diaphragm to get a hole or a tear in it.

» Some women find that a cervical cap is more difficult to put in place or remove than a diaphragm.

» If you find that the cervical cap has moved out of place during sex, you may want to use emergency contraception.

» Oil-based products should not be used with cervical caps because they can damage the latex rubber.

SPERMICIDES

Most authorities don't recommend that you use spermicide by itself because it may not be very effective. You can use it as a backup with condoms or diaphragms if you want to, but some studies show it doesn't increase their effectiveness. You may find that is it difficult to buy spermicide in Australia at present.

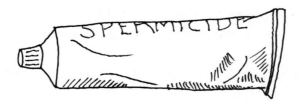

Spermicide

What is spermicide?

Spermicide is a type of cream or gel with chemicals in it that kill sperm. The spermicide that is available in Australia comes in a tube about the same size as a tube of toothpaste (see illustration above). It has an applicator, or introducer, like a plastic tube with a plunger, that you use to insert the spermicide right back at the far end of your vagina, so that it is as close to the opening in the cervix as possible.

Are there different kinds of spermicide?

There are quite a few different kinds of spermicide available in other countries, but in Australia we only have one, which is a water-based gel. Its trade name is Gynol II®.

How does spermicide work?

When it's used correctly, spermicide forms a barrier at the opening of the cervix and kills any sperm that come into contact with it. If the spermicide works, sperm die before they can travel up the fallopian tubes to meet an egg, so you don't get pregnant.

How effective is spermicide?

There are no good figures on the effectiveness of spermicide used by itself. Some studies have shown that it may be only 60 per cent effective.

Why would I want to choose spermicide?

You may want to use spermicide with a condom or a diaphragm if you think that you would feel safer from getting pregnant if you use it as well. You don't need a doctor's prescription, and anyone can buy it.

You may want to have a tube of spermicide and an applicator handy as a backup in an emergency, for example if you found that your diaphragm had a hole in it or your condom had torn or come off. But you should know that if you put spermicide in after the man has come, it can only work on the sperm still in the vagina. It has no effect on the sperm that have already gone up through the opening in the cervix and into the uterus. Still, it can be worth trying in an absolute emergency because the less live sperm around, the less chance there is of one fertilising an egg. But remember that emergency contraception is much more effective in this type of situation.

HOW DO I USE SPERMICIDE?

Using spermicide on its own

1   Take the cap off the tube and screw on the applicator in its place.

2   Squeeze the tube until the applicator is full of gel, and the plunger has been pushed out as far as it will go.

3   Unscrew the applicator from the tube.

4   Leave the plunger as it is, pushed out.

5   Gently slide the applicator into your vagina. It is best if you are lying down with your knees bent, or crouching down or if you have one foot up on a chair or on the toilet or the bath.

6   Ease the applicator in as far as you can. Don't worry, it can't get lost inside you. It can only go as far as the end of your vagina, and it cannot fit into the opening in your cervix because that opening is much smaller than the applicator.

7   Push the plunger right in slowly so that all the gel comes out into your vagina.

8   Slide the applicator out of your vagina.

9   Wait a few minutes for the spermicide to spread itself around inside your vagina.

10   Now you can have sex.

Using spermicide with a diaphragm

If you are using the spermicide with a diaphragm, it is very important that the spermicide is water-based, like Gynol II®. Check the package to be sure you can use it safely with a diaphragm.

Squeeze about a teaspoon of spermicide into the bowl of the diaphragm. It needs to go on the side closest to your cervix. Try not to get any on the rim, because this will make the diaphragm very slippery and difficult to hold. Insert the diaphragm with the spermicide on it.

Using spermicide with a condom

If you are using spermicide with a condom, the spermicide should be water-based. Check the package to be sure. Use the applicator and put the spermicide directly into the vagina as discussed.

Most spermicides are only effective for about one hour, so they should be used as close to the time you have sex as possible. After you have had sex, wash the applicator with soap and water. Make sure you wash the inside as well as the outside. Keep it somewhere clean and dry.

Where do I get spermicide?

You can buy spermicide from some chemists, or online.

What does it cost?

Spermicide costs about $18.

Frequently asked questions about spermicide

Q Does spermicide have any side effects?

A Very few people are allergic to spermicide, but those who are allergic usually feel itchy or sore. It is best to go to a doctor to be checked if the symptoms don't stop in a few hours because you might have an infection rather than an allergy.

Q If I use spermicide with my diaphragm, and my partner comes and then we start again, should I put an applicator of spermicide in before he comes again?

A No, it isn't necessary.

Things to think about if you are considering spermicide

» Remember that spermicide by itself can be unreliable. When it is used by itself it must be inserted very close to the opening in your cervix for it to work best and even if you manage to put it there, your body heat makes it melt and it can run out of your vagina easily.

» You have to remember to have it with you if you think you may have sex when you are not at home.

» If spermicide is the only contraception you are prepared to use, it is better to use it than to use nothing at all, just as long as you are aware of the risk. This would be the time to really consider what you would do if you had an unplanned pregnancy, so you could be prepared if it happened.

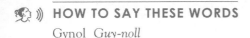 **HOW TO SAY THESE WORDS**

Gynol *Guy-noll*

3

THE CONTRACEPTIVE PILL

I'm sure you will have heard about the contraceptive pill. It is a very popular method of contraception. There are basically two kinds of contraceptive pill. They both contain hormones that are chemicals, similar to the ones produced in your body to regulate your reproductive system.

One kind of contraceptive pill combines two hormones, oestrogen and progestogen. It is called the combined oral contraceptive pill. The other kind contains only one of these hormones, progestogen. It is called the progestogen-only pill or the minipill.

In this first session we will just talk about the combined oral contraceptive pill and because it is used more often, it is generally just called 'the Pill', so that's what we will call it too.

THE PILL
(THE COMBINED ORAL CONTRACEPTIVE PILL)

What is the Pill?

The Pill is exactly what its name tells us. It is a little pill containing hormones that can act in your body to prevent pregnancy. Sometimes the Pill comes in a pack of just 21 hormone pills. The pills come packed in a foil sheet in little plastic bubbles, with the days written underneath so that you can easily see where you are up to. With 21-day pills you take a pill every day for 21 days and then take a week long break between packs before you start again.

The Pill also comes in packs of 28 pills. Depending on the type of pill, they have either 21 or 24 hormone pills. The other pills in the pack have no hormones in them, but they are there so that you get into the habit of taking a pill every single day. Those extra pills, which are a different colour in the pack so you can recognise them, are sometimes called dummy pills or sugar pills. They help a lot if you are inclined to forget about starting the next pack at the right time. With both types of packs you will have a period during the days without hormone pills.

Are there different types of the Pill?

The combined oral contraceptive pill comes in two different types of formula. They are called monophasic and triphasic formulas and they vary as follows:

» Monophasic pills have exactly the same oestrogen and progestogen dose in each of the pills.

» Triphasic pills have more oestrogen in the middle of the pack, and the progestogen is increased twice during the course of the pack. Each different type of pill will be a different colour in the pack.

With both formulas there are pills that have different combinations of the two hormones. But they all work in the same way to prevent pregnancy.

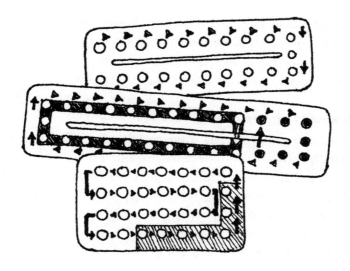

The Pill (the combined oral contraceptive pill)

How does the Pill work?

The oestrogen and the progestogen taken together each day prevent the ovaries from releasing an egg. The progestogen also makes the mucus in the cervix thicker so that sperm cannot get through and makes the lining of the uterus thinner so that even if an egg were fertilised, it cannot implant and grow there.

How effective is the Pill?

If you take the Pill every day as directed, it can be over 99 per cent effective. This means that if 100 women used the Pill as their method of contraception for a year, no more than one of them, and perhaps none of them, would have an unplanned pregnancy.

But because we are only human and humans make mistakes, the Pill is not always taken as directed. Sometimes women forget to take their pills, and if they don't take them as directed they are more likely to get pregnant. So it is more accurate to say that between one and eight of the women who used the Pill for a year would have an unplanned pregnancy.

Why would I want to choose the Pill?

The main reason you may want to take the Pill is that you absolutely do not want to be pregnant, and it is one of the most effective methods of contraception. Another reason could be that because you take the Pill every day, you do not have to think about contraception when you are going to have sex.

Are there any side effects to using the Pill?

Many women do get some side effects from the Pill for the first couple of months, but they usually settle down after about three months. Some common side effects are breakthrough bleeding or spotting between periods, headache, sore breasts and nausea. You may find that spotting between periods will improve if you are careful to take the Pill at the same time every day.

Some of the less common side effects include putting on weight, less desire for sex and feeling irritable. But these could also be caused by other things happening in your life and might have nothing to do with taking the Pill. So if any of these things happen to you, talk to a doctor or nurse to find out what is causing your symptoms. Then you can decide how to deal with it.

If one type of the Pill does give you unwanted side effects, don't just put up with it. Tell your doctor. There are other types of the Pill you can try, and you should be able to find one that suits you.

Are there any reasons why I could not use the Pill?

You cannot use the Pill if you have had a deep vein thrombosis, which is a blood clot in a vein, or if you have had a stroke or heart attack. You cannot take it if you have severe liver problems, focal migraine (which is a special severe kind of migraine) or uncontrolled high blood pressure.

If you have any unusual bleeding from your vagina that hasn't been diagnosed then you will have to wait until you know what is causing it before you can take the Pill. You will probably not be able to take the Pill if you have cancer in your breast, uterus or ovary, because the hormones in the Pill can affect the cancer, and could make it spread.

If you are breastfeeding and you want to keep breastfeeding then you won't be able to use the combined oral contraceptive pill because the oestrogen reduces milk production, but you can probably take the minipill or one of the other hormonal types of contraception that doesn't contain any oestrogen.

Are there any other things that could cause a problem if I want to take the Pill?

You may not be able to take the Pill if any of the following things apply to you. If you have common migraine, diabetes, are being treated for tuberculosis (TB), have a strong family history of thrombosis (blood clots in veins) or severe depression then you will need to talk it over with your doctor.

If you are taking other medications, you should also tell your doctor in case they could react with the Pill and make it less effective. If you are over 35 and smoke, or you are under 35 and smoke more than 15 cigarettes a day, this should be discussed too. If there is a chance you could be pregnant, you will probably need to wait until you can have a pregnancy test to be sure you are not pregnant before you start the Pill.

HOW DO I USE THE PILL?

You should start on the first pack of pills when you have a period. Read the instructions on the pack to find out exactly what to do for the type of Pill you have. Ask your doctor if it will work straightaway or if you need to use another type of contraceptive, like condoms, if you have sex during the first seven days when you take the Pill for the very first time. You may want to use condoms whenever you have sex even though you are on the Pill, because condoms help to protect you from sexually transmissible infections (STIs).

Anyway, once you start taking the Pill, if you have a 28-day pack, you just keep taking a pill every day. If you have a 21 day pack, when you finish all the pills you have to wait seven days and then start a new pack.

What happens if I miss a pill?

If you miss taking a pill, but you remember within 24 hours, take the pill as soon as you remember. Take the next pill at the usual time. You will still be covered for contraception.

If it is more than 24 hours since you should have taken a pill, take one as soon as you remember and take the next pill at the usual time. Keep taking a pill every day, but it will be seven days before you are fully covered for contraception, so if you have sex during the next seven days it's best to use condoms or another method of contraception, as well. You can ring a Family Planning centre or your doctor if you feel worried. It's better to be absolutely sure what to do, than to wait and see what happens.

Where do I get the Pill?

You need to go to your doctor or a Family Planning centre or Sexual Health clinic to get a prescription for the Pill. This is important because you need to have a check-up and talk to a doctor or nurse to see which type of the Pill will suit you best. You can see a doctor and buy the Pill at a Family Planning centre. If you go to another doctor, you take the prescription and buy your Pill from a chemist.

What does the Pill cost?

Prices vary but for Pills that are listed on the Pharmaceutical Benefits Scheme (PBS) it is usually about $5 to $6 for a packet that lasts for one month, and about $30 per one-month packet for those that are not listed. If you have a Pharmaceutical Concession Card, PBS-listed Pills will cost less but there is no reduction in price for Pills not listed on the PBS.

Frequently asked questions about the Pill

Q If I take the Pill every day just as it says on the pack, how could I get pregnant accidentally?

A The Pill is not 100 per cent effective even if it is taken exactly as directed. Also, if you are sick then you could lose the effects of the Pill by vomiting or having diarrhoea before it had a chance to work. If you do vomit or have diarrhoea it would be best to follow the instructions for missed pills to be sure you are protected.

Another thing to watch for is that some antibiotics and other medications, and even natural therapies, may react with the Pill and stop it from working. You really need to talk to your doctor about this. If you have to see a different doctor for any reason, tell her or him that you are taking the Pill, so you are not given medication that could react with it.

Q If I want to get pregnant, can I stop taking the Pill and get pregnant right away?

A It takes the average woman about six months of trying to get pregnant even if she's not taking the Pill and maybe a couple of months extra if she has been on the Pill. The problem is that this is an average. Some women get pregnant in the first month after they stop taking the Pill, and some perfectly normal women will still not be pregnant after 12 months of trying. If your periods aren't back to normal after three or four months, or if you have been trying to get pregnant for more than twelve months, see your doctor or Family Planning centre for advice.

Q What if I miss a period when I'm taking the Pill?

A You may miss a period while you are on the Pill. This is common and is usually nothing to worry about. As long as you have been taking the pills as directed, just keep taking them as usual. If you miss a second period then see your doctor or Family Planning centre for advice.

Q Since I started taking the Pill, my periods have been really short, and only last a few days and there hasn't been much blood. The colour is darker too. Is this OK?

A This is quite normal and happens to most women when they are taking the Pill.

Q Should I have any special check-ups when I am on the Pill?

A It's a good idea to have your blood pressure taken, and to discuss any physical changes each time you go for a new prescription for the Pill. Also be aware of the way your breasts look and feel and tell your doctor if you notice any changes. You should have a Pap test every two years, and sometimes more often if your Pap tests have been abnormal in the past.

Q I know of someone who got brown blotches on her skin when she was sunbaking after she started taking the Pill. Is this common?

A No, it isn't common, but it can happen. These types of blotches are called chloasma, and are caused by an uneven skin response to the sun because of the oestrogen in the Pill. Once you are on the Pill it's good to wear a hat and use an SPF (sun protection factor) 15+ sunscreen on any exposed skin if you're out in the sun. If you get this skin reaction and it becomes a problem for you, the minipill (or other methods of contraception that don't contain oestrogen) may suit you better.

Q I have to have an operation and a friend told me I'll have to stop taking the Pill before I go to hospital. Is that true?

A Yes, it probably is. You need to talk to your doctor as soon as possible because most women are asked to stop taking the Pill from between four to six weeks before they have surgery. If you do have to stop taking it, remember to use other contraception, like condoms, if you have sex. You should also stop taking the Pill if you have to stay in bed for a long time, or you have a leg in plaster. This is because if you are not moving around normally, there is a risk that you could get blood clots in your veins.

Things to think about if you are considering using the Pill

» The main thing to think about if you decide to use the Pill is that you must remember to take it every day. If you are not going to be at home when you usually take your pill, you must remember to take it with you.

» It is very important that you go to a doctor to get the Pill prescribed. It can be dangerous to take a Pill that has been prescribed for someone else. Everyone should be checked first and then given the type of Pill that will suit them best.

» Even if you use the Pill for contraception, you may want to use condoms as well because they help to protect you against sexually transmissible infections (STIs).

 ## HOW TO SAY THESE WORDS

chloasma *klo-az-ma*

diarrhoea *die-are-ee-ah*

hormones *hor-moans*

monophasic *mon-no-fay-zick*

oestrogen *ee-stra-jen*

progestogen *pro-jest-a-jen*

triphasic *try-fay-zick*

THE MINIPILL (THE PROGESTOGEN-ONLY PILL)

Now we'll talk about the minipill. It isn't quite as effective as the combined pill so it is not used as often in Australia.

What is the minipill?

The minipill is the name most people use when they are talking about the progestogen-only pill (see illustration opposite). This type of pill contains only one hormone, progestogen, and you may also hear the minipill called the POP, which is short for progestogen-only pill.

You have to take the minipill every single day without a break, and every pill is a hormone pill. There are no dummy or sugar pills in a minipill pack. It is also important to take the minipill at the same time every day. All minipills come in packs of 28 pills, and all the pills have the same dose of hormone in them.

Are there different types of the minipill?

There are four brands of minipill available in Australia, but they all contain one of two kinds of the hormone progestogen. Some women might find that one kind of minipill suits them really well while the other one gives them problems.

How does the minipill work?

The progestogen in the minipill acts in your body to make the mucus in your cervix thicker, so that the sperm can't get through. It also causes changes in the lining of the uterus so that even if an egg were fertilised, it cannot implant in the lining and grow there. In many women progestogen can also

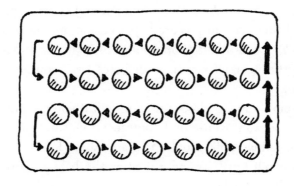

The minipill

stop the ovaries from releasing an egg every month. But some women still release an egg and have normal periods just as if they weren't taking the minipill at all.

How effective is the minipill?

The minipill is 92 to 99.7 per cent effective. This means that if 100 women used the minipill as their method of contraception for one year, somewhere between none and eight of them would have an unplanned pregnancy. As with most other methods, if you use it correctly every day it will be much more effective. If you don't remember to take the minipill at the same time every day, you will be very much at risk of having an unplanned pregnancy.

Women who are breastfeeding or women who are older and don't ovulate as often generally find the minipill most effective.

Why would I want to choose the minipill?

The minipill could be a good choice for you if you are not able to take oestrogen, or you get side effects that worry you when you take oestrogen. An advantage of the minipill is that you can take it even if you have some medical conditions that prevent you from taking the combined oral contraceptive pill. A few of these conditions are hypertension, migraines or liver disease. You can take the minipill even if you have had blood clots in the veins, if you have diabetes, or if you are over 35 and smoke.

You may want to choose the minipill if you are breastfeeding and you want to use oral contraception, since progestogen does not reduce milk supply. You are advised not to take the combined pill until six months after the baby is born if you are breastfeeding, because the oestrogen in it will reduce your milk supply.

Some women will get brown marks on their face when they take the combined Pill and go out in the sun. This does not happen to women on the minipill, though if they have taken the combined pill first, and got brown marks, the marks may still take many months to fade completely. Some women just like the idea of using a hormonal method of contraception that is fairly effective but has less hormones in it than a combined pill.

Are there any side effects with the minipill?

The most common side effect of the minipill is that periods often become irregular. The time between periods can be shorter or longer than usual. You could even find that your periods disappear altogether. You could also have spotting in between periods.

Some women may get headaches or sore breasts. Some women put on weight because the progestogen in the mini-pill increases their appetite and they eat more, but this is not very common because of the very low dose of hormones in the minipill. Some women don't have any side effects at all.

Are there any reasons why I could not use the minipill?

There are very few women who shouldn't ever take the mini-pill. There are also some things you should talk over with your doctor before you decide to use it. If you have unusual bleed-ing from your vagina that hasn't been diagnosed, or if there is any chance you could be pregnant, both these issues need to be sorted out before you start taking the minipill. You should also tell your doctor if you have liver disease, breast cancer or a disease of your ovaries, or you are taking medication for epilepsy, TB or HIV/AIDS.

Are there any other things that could cause a problem if I take the minipill?

If you have any illness that causes you to vomit or have diarrhoea, you should talk about this too. And tell your doctor if you are on any medication in case it could react with the minipill. But don't worry, antibiotics don't lower the effectiveness of the minipill.

There is some evidence that if you weigh more than 70 kilograms then the usual dose of the minipill may not be as effective, but you can ask your doctor if this is an issue.

What do I do if I miss a minipill?

If you miss taking a minipill, take the next pill as soon as you remember it, and take the following pill at the usual time. If you are more than three hours late taking your pill, and you have sex during the next two days, you should use condoms or another form of contraception.

If you miss pills around the time that you have unprotected sex, you may want to think about using emergency contraception. You can ring a Family Planning centre or your doctor if you feel worried. It's better to be absolutely sure what to do than to wait and see what happens.

Where do I get the minipill?

You have to go to a local doctor or see a doctor at a Family Planning centre to have the minipill prescribed for you. The doctor will take your medical history and give you a check-up that will include taking your weight and blood pressure and possibly a Pap test if this is due.

HOW DO I USE THE MINIPILL?

You must take the minipill at the same time every day for it to work effectively. Choose a time that will suit you to take it every day from then on and take the very first pill at that time on the first day of your period.

The minipill works best to prevent pregnancy between 3 and 21 hours after you have taken each pill. It's a good idea to work out the best time to take it so that you will be fully covered if you have sex. If you usually have sex at night, or first thing in the morning, then the best time to take the minipill would be at lunchtime or early in the evening. Just swallow the pill with water.

The minipill comes in a pack of 28 pills, so when you've finished one pack just start straightaway on the next pack. You don't have any break from taking the pills.

If you are not having periods, for example if you are breastfeeding, and your periods haven't returned since the baby was born, you can start taking the minipill whenever you like.

It is important to use other contraception, like condoms, if you have sex during the next seven days after you first start the minipill, to make sure you are covered against pregnancy.

Keep on taking the minipill until you decide that you want to use another type of contraception or you want to get pregnant.

What does the minipill cost?

Prices vary but a packet of minipills that lasts for one month costs about $5 on the Pharmaceutical Benefits Scheme (PBS). It costs even less if you have a Pharmaceutical Concessions Card.

Frequently asked questions about the minipill

Q I am on the minipill and often forget to take my pill when I am supposed to. I haven't got pregnant, though, so does it really matter?

A If you really don't want to be pregnant then it does matter. Even though you have not become pregnant so far, you could get pregnant any time that you are late taking the minipill if you have sex around that time. Perhaps you could choose another time to take your pill when you are most likely to remember it.

If you are often late taking your pills or you miss a pill at least once every month, you are at a much higher risk of getting pregnant. It would be best to consider changing to another method of contraception that will be more reliable for you.

Q I only missed one minipill and now my period is overdue. Should I have a pregnancy test or am I worrying too much?

A Even though you only missed one pill it is possible you could be pregnant if you have had sex since you missed the pill. Irregular periods are very common on the minipill even if you're not pregnant but it's probably better to know for certain if there's any chance at all. A urine pregnancy test is simple and accurate.

Q If I got pregnant when I missed one of my minipills, but I didn't know I was pregnant so I kept taking the pills, would that affect the baby?

A There is no evidence that the minipill has any bad effects on an unborn baby.

Q Do I need to have regular check-ups if I take the minipill?

A It's a good idea to have your blood pressure taken each time that you go for a new prescription for the minipill. Be aware of how your breasts look and feel, and tell your doctor if you notice any changes. You should also have a Pap test every two years, or more often sometimes, if you have had an abnormal Pap test in the past.

Things to think about if you are considering using the minipill

» If you decide to use the minipill, it is very important that you remember to take it every day and at the same time every day. If you are not going to be at home when you usually take your pill, you must remember to take it with you.

» It is very important that you go to a doctor to get your own prescription for the minipill. It can be dangerous to take a pill that has been prescribed for someone else. Everyone should be checked first and then given the type of pill that will suit them best.

» If you use the minipill for contraception then you may want to use condoms as well because they help to protect you against sexually transmissible infections (STIs).

 HOW TO SAY THESE WORDS

cycts *sists*

ectopic *eck-top-ick*

4

VAGINAL RINGS

THE VAGINAL RING

What is a vaginal ring?

The vaginal ring is a new method of contraception. It is a soft, thin, doughnut-like ring of silastic, which is a type of plastic, containing hormones. The vaginal ring is placed in the vagina to prevent pregnancy.

Are there different types of vaginal rings?

There is only one type of vaginal ring available in Australia. Like the combined oral contraceptive pill, it contains two hormones, oestrogen and progestogen, so it is called a combined vaginal ring. Its trade name is NuvaRing®. As it is the only type of vaginal ring we have at present, we will just call it 'the vaginal ring'.

How does the vaginal ring work?

Instead of having to take a pill every day, the hormones in the vaginal ring are slowly released into the woman's body through the skin in her vagina.

How effective is the vaginal ring?

The combined vaginal ring is as effective as the combined oral contraceptive pill, and if it is used correctly it can be more than 99 per cent effective. This means that if 100 women used the vaginal ring for a year, less than one of them would have an unplanned pregnancy. But because people sometimes make mistakes, the vaginal ring is not always used correctly, so it is more accurate to say that if 100 women used the vaginal ring for a year, up to eight of them might have an unplanned pregnancy.

Why would I want to choose the vaginal ring?

A vaginal ring could be suitable for you if you like the Pill because it is so reliable but have trouble remembering to take it every day. It could be an alternative for those women who find it hard to swallow tablets. The vaginal ring could be a good alternative if you have an illness that stops you absorbing medications through your digestive system. If you take the Pill and the hormones are not absorbed into your body very well, the hormone level may not be high enough to stop a pregnancy from happening. With the vaginal ring, the hormones do not go through the digestive system, but are absorbed into your body through your vagina.

Are there any side effects to using the vaginal ring?

Many women do get some side effects from the vaginal ring at first, but they usually settle down after about three months. Some common side effects are breakthrough bleeding or spotting between periods, sore breasts, nausea, and vaginal irritation and discharge.

Some of the less common side effects include putting on weight, less desire for sex and feeling irritable. But these could

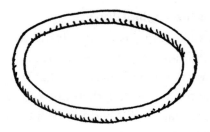

The vaginal ring

also be caused by other things happening in your life and might have nothing to do with using the vaginal ring. So if any of these things happen to you, talk to a doctor or nurse to find out what is causing your symptoms. Then you can decide how to deal with it.

Are there any reasons why I could not use the vaginal ring?
Similar to taking the combined oral contraceptive pill, you cannot use the combined vaginal ring if you have had a deep vein thrombosis, which is a blood clot in a vein, or if you have had a stroke or a heart attack. You cannot use it if you have severe liver problems, focal migraine, which is a special severe kind of migraine, or uncontrolled high blood pressure.

If you have any unusual bleeding from your vagina that hasn't been diagnosed then you will have to wait until you know what is causing it before you can use the vaginal ring. You will probably not be able to use the vaginal ring if you have had cancer in your breast, uterus or ovary.

If you are breastfeeding and you want to keep breastfeeding, you won't be able to use the vaginal ring until six months after the birth because the oestrogen reduces milk supply. You can probably take the minipill or one of the other hormonal types of contraception that doesn't contain any oestrogen.

HOW DO I USE THE VAGINAL RING?

You can insert your first ring sometime between the first day of a period and the fifth day after your period starts. You could also start using the vaginal ring at any time if you're absolutely sure that you are not pregnant, but if you do start using it after the fifth day from when your period began, you will need to use another method as well (like condoms) for seven days.

You put the vaginal ring high up inside your vagina. It doesn't fit around the cervix, it just lies in the vagina. To put it in comfortably, you just squeeze it across the middle so that it slides into your vagina easily, like a tampon. Once you have put it into your vagina you do not need to keep taking it out and putting it back in. You do not need to remember to use the vaginal ring when you have sex because it is already in place. Some women may prefer to take it out before they have sex and put it back in soon afterwards. That is fine but it is not necessary, and it must not be left out for more than three hours.

The vaginal ring stays in place in your vagina for three weeks. Then you take it out and have seven days break from using it, just as you would if you were taking dummy pills in the combined oral contraceptive pill pack. During the break, you will have a period. After seven days, you put a new vaginal ring in your vagina for another three weeks, and so on, as long as you are happy to keep using it.

If you want to avoid having a period at any time, you can leave the ring in place for three to four weeks and when you remove it, insert a new one immediately. It is best to check with your doctor about this.

You may not be able to use the vaginal ring if any of the following things apply to you. If you have common migraine, diabetes, are being treated for tuberculosis (TB), have a strong family history of thrombosis (blood clots in veins), or severe depression then you will need to talk it over with your doctor.

If you are taking other medications then you should also tell your doctor in case they react with the hormones in the vaginal ring and make it less effective. If you are over 35 and smoke or you are under 35 and smoke more than 15 cigarettes a day, this should be discussed too. If there is a chance you could be pregnant, you will probably need to wait until you can have a pregnancy test to be sure you are not pregnant before you start using the vaginal ring.

What if I forget to take the vaginal ring out at the right time?
If your vaginal ring has been left in for between three and four weeks, take it out and insert a new ring 28 days after your last ring was inserted. This may mean you have a very short ring-free break, but that is alright and you will still be covered for contraception.

If your vaginal ring has been left in for more than four weeks, take it out, insert a new ring right away, and use condoms for the next seven days. If you have had unprotected sex in the last five days, you should consider using emergency contraception as well.

What if I forget to insert a new vaginal ring at the right time?
If you are less than 24 hours late inserting a new ring, don't worry, you're still covered for contraception.

If you are more than 24 hours late inserting a new ring, insert a new ring right away, and use condoms for the next seven days. If you have had unprotected sex in the last five days, you should consider using emergency contraception as well.

Where do I get the vaginal ring?

You can get a prescription and buy the vaginal ring at Family Planning centres. You can also see a local doctor for a prescription and then buy your vaginal ring from a chemist.

What does the vaginal ring cost?

A vaginal ring costs about $80 for three rings from a chemist, and $25 for one and $65 for three rings from Family Planning centres.

Frequently asked questions about the vaginal ring

Q If I take the vaginal ring out when I have sex, how long can I leave it out and still be covered for contraception?

A You must put it back in within three hours.

Q What if I forget and leave the vaginal ring out for a long time?

A If you forget and leave it out for longer than three hours, put it back in as soon as you remember and use condoms for the next seven days.

If this happens between the first and seventh day of using that vaginal ring, and you have had unprotected sex in the five days before you left the ring out, you should consider using emergency contraception as well.

If it happens between the 15th and 21st day of using the ring, just keep using that ring until it is due to be removed, then insert a new ring immediately without having a ring-free break.

Q Can I use a vaginal ring as soon as I have had a baby?

A No, vaginal rings should not be used for the first three weeks after a baby is born, because of the higher risk of the hormones in the ring causing blood clotting during that time. Three weeks after the birth you can use the vaginal ring if you are not breastfeeding.

Q Can I use the vaginal ring if I am breastfeeding?

A The vaginal ring is not recommended if you are breastfeeding a baby less than six months old. After six months, if your baby is having other food as well as breast milk, you can use the vaginal ring.

Q Do I need to have regular check-ups if I am using a vaginal ring?

A Yes, you will need to go to your doctor for a check-up four months after you start using the vaginal ring, and then once a year while you are still using it.

Things to think about if you are considering the vaginal ring

» You need to notice that the vaginal ring has not come out accidentally, such as when you take out a tampon.

» The vaginal ring does not protect you from sexually transmissible infections (STIs) so you may want to use condoms as well.

HOW TO SAY THESE WORDS

NuvaRing® *Noovar ring*

5

INJECTABLE HORMONAL CONTRACEPTION (THE INJECTION)

PROGESTOGEN-ONLY INJECTIONS (DMPA)

In this session, we will discuss the progestogen-only injection. You will probably have heard of it by one of its trade names, either Depo-Provera® or Depo-Ralovera®. To make it easier to talk about, we will call it DMPA. DMPA stands for depot medroxyprogesterone acetate, which is the type of progestogen that is used in this kind of injection.

What is DMPA?

DMPA is a liquid that contains the hormone progestogen, similar to the progestogen in the progestogen-only pill. It is given as an injection into the muscle of your arm or buttocks. When people are talking about injectable hormonal contraception they sometimes just call DMPA 'the Injection'.

The most important thing about DMPA is that it stays in your body and keeps working to stop you getting pregnant for three months at a time.

Are there different types of DMPA?

At the moment there is only one kind of hormone injection that you can get in Australia. The same injection is available under two different trade names, Depo-Provera® and Depo-Ralovera®.

How does DMPA work?

DMPA stops a woman's ovaries from releasing eggs. It makes the mucus in the opening of the cervix thicker, so sperm cannot get through, and it changes the lining of the uterus so if by some chance an egg were fertilised, it couldn't grow there.

How effective is DMPA?

DMPA is 97 to 99.7 per cent effective, which means it is really very effective. If 100 women used DMPA as their method of contraception for a year, no more than three of them, and perhaps none of them, would have an unplanned pregnancy.

Why would I want to choose DMPA?

You may want to use DMPA if you definitely don't want to become pregnant and you have tried the Pill but keep forgetting to take it. You may have already had an unplanned pregnancy after forgetting to take the Pill. You may want to use DMPA if you think that you will find it hard to take the Pill every day, and you really don't want to risk an unplanned pregnancy. Perhaps you just don't want to have to remember to use contraception all the time, and you think having an injection every three months would be easier. You might think about trying DMPA if you cannot use contraception containing oestrogen for health reasons or if you get problem side effects from it. You can use DMPA safely when you are breastfeeding.

Are there any reasons why I could not use DMPA?

You cannot use DMPA if there is any chance you could be pregnant. You may be advised not to use it if you have breast cancer or any breast problems that have not yet been diagnosed. If you have a medical problem that prevents you from having an injection into your muscles, you will not be able to have DMPA.

If you have any medical conditions, you should let your doctor know before you use DMPA, just to make sure it will not cause problems.

Does DMPA have any side effects?

The main side effect of DMPA is that women's periods usually change. Periods are more likely to get lighter, but they occasionally get heavier and they can become quite irregular. You may have a bit of spotting between periods. You may stop bleeding altogether after a few injections. This is okay and will not harm you. Some women also gain weight or have headaches or feel depressed. If this happens to you, see your doctor.

HOW DO I USE DMPA?

The best time to have the first injection of DMPA is during the first five days of your menstrual cycle. You count a menstrual cycle from the first day of a period until the first day of the next period. Count the first day of your period as day one. Any day between then and day five, the fifth day, is a good time to start. This is because you can be fairly sure you are not pregnant. But really, you can start on DMPA at any time if you are absolutely sure you are not pregnant and you are happy to use another method of contraception as backup for seven days after you have the first injection.

Where do I get DMPA?

You need to go to a doctor to get an injection of DMPA. You can go to your local doctor or to a doctor at a Family Planning centre. The doctor will talk to you and examine you, and then they will either give you a prescription for you to take to the chemist or, if they have DMPA at the surgery, give you the injection straightaway. If you have to buy it from a chemist then you will need to go back to the doctor to have the injection.

What does it cost?

DMPA costs about $17 every 12 weeks on the Australian Pharmaceutical Benefits Scheme (PBS). It costs even less if you have a Health Care Card.

Frequently asked questions about DMPA

Q Does it hurt?

A Not usually. It's a very small injection and most people find it doesn't hurt much at all.

Q What if I am late going back for my next injection?

A If it is less than two weeks from the date that you were due to have the repeat injection, you can have another injection and you should be covered against pregnancy. If it is more than two weeks after the date that you were due to have the repeat injection, and you have had sex in those two weeks, you may have to wait a while to make sure you are not pregnant. Ask your doctor about this.

Use condoms or the minipill for three weeks from the last time you had sex, and then have a pregnancy test. If the test is negative, which means you are not pregnant, you can have another injection. If the test is positive, which means you are pregnant, talk to your doctor about the choices you have.

Q If I want to become pregnant when I stop having the injections, will it be more difficult for me to get pregnant because I have been using DMPA for a long time?

A No, it does not matter how long you have been using DMPA, it would take you the same length of time to get pregnant as it would take if you had used it only once. It is true, though, that it can take quite a long time for a regular period pattern to start after you stop using DMPA. Eight months to a year is not unusual.

Q I've heard that DMPA can make you infertile. Is that true?

A No. Once your periods come back, your chances of pregnancy are the same as they were before you started it. But because of the long delay, it probably isn't a great choice for someone who is thinking about starting a family in the next year or two.

Q Does DMPA increase my chances of getting breast cancer?

A DMPA was found to increase the risk of breast cancer in some of the experimental animals in which it was first tried. There is absolutely no evidence that it increases the risk of breast cancer in women.

Things to think about if you are considering using DMPA

» Once you have the injection, you will have the effect of DMPA in your system for three months. You cannot do anything to stop it or take it away. So while you are covered for contraception for three months, you will also have any side effects for those three months.

» After you stop having injections of DMPA, it may take up to 12 months before your periods return to normal.

» If you stop having injections of DMPA and you want to become pregnant, it may take a while, though most women will become pregnant within two years.

» If you stop having injections of DMPA and you don't want to be pregnant, you should use another method of contraception right away. Some women become pregnant very quickly after stopping DMPA.

» DMPA does not protect a woman from sexually transmissible infections (STIs). You may want to think about using condoms as well as DMPA because condoms help to protect you from STIs.

HOW TO SAY THESE WORDS

acetate *assy-tate*

Depot medroxyprogesterone *Deppo med-rock-see-pro-jest-a-roan*

Depo-Provera® *Deppo Pro-vera*

Depo-Ralovera® *Deppo Ral-owe-vera*

6

IMPLANTS

PROGESTOGEN-ONLY IMPLANTS

The contraceptive implant is a relatively new way of using hormonal contraception. As you can imagine, an implant is meant to be a fairly long-term method of contraception, so some women find it a great alternative to other methods.

What is an implant?

A contraceptive implant is a little plastic rod or a set of rods containing hormones that are inserted just underneath the skin, usually on the inside of the upper arm. The hormones are released into your body over a period of time and prevent you from becoming pregnant.

Are there different types of implants?

The only implant available in Australia at present is a progestogen-only implant. Its trade name is Implanon® (page 74). It is a small, single, flexible plastic rod, about 4 centimetres long and only 2 millimetres thick. It contains progestogen inside a special coating that stops the hormone being released

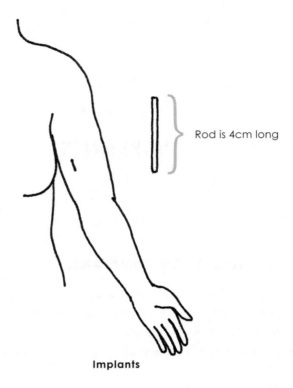

Rod is 4cm long

Implants

all at once. The progestogen is slowly released into the woman's body over a period of about three years. For this session we will call it 'the Implant'.

How does the Implant work?

Progestogen-only implants make the mucus in the cervix thicker so that sperm cannot get through into the uterus and up into the fallopian tubes to fertilise an egg. They also cause changes in the lining of the uterus so that even if an egg were fertilised it could not implant and grow there. The progestogen in Implanon® also stops the ovaries from releasing an egg each month.

How effective is the Implant?

Implanon® is more than 99 per cent effective. This means that if 100 women used this type of implant as their method of contraception for one year, at most only one woman would have an unplanned pregnancy.

Why would I want to choose the Implant?

You may want to have the Implant if you need a very effective method of contraception that you don't have to think about every day or remember to use. If you don't want to be pregnant for a couple of years or more, but you would like a method of contraception that can be easily reversed, the Implant may be a good choice. If you are not able to take the hormone oestrogen, or you get unwanted side effects from it, you may find that using a method of contraception that has no oestrogen in it, like a progestogen-only implant, suits you.

Are there any reasons I could not have the Implant?

You would not be able to have an implant if there is a chance you could be pregnant. If you have unusual bleeding from your vagina that hasn't been diagnosed, you shouldn't have an implant until the reason for the bleeding is known. Hormonal problems or a history of hormone-affected cancers, like breast cancer, may mean you can't use the Implant for contraception. You would need to discuss this with your doctor. A few medications can react with the progestogen in the Implant and may make it less effective at preventing a pregnancy. Tell your doctor if you are taking any medication and find out if you can still have the Implant.

HOW IS THE IMPLANT INSERTED?

Most doctors will ask you to make two appointments, one to decide whether an implant is a good choice for you, and the other to have it inserted at the right time in the cycle. If you decide to have it inserted and it happens to be the right time in the cycle, some doctors may be happy to insert it on the same day after you have collected the Implant from the chemist.

It takes about one minute to insert Implanon®. The doctor will put a small mark on your skin on the inside of your upper arm. The skin will be cleaned with antiseptic and a little local anaesthetic will be injected into the area so that it goes numb. The injection might sting a bit, but after that the insertion will be quite comfortable. When the area is numb, the doctor will insert an introducer just under your skin. The introducer is a thin tube containing the Implant. The doctor uses the introducer to put the Implant in the right place. When the introducer is carefully pulled away, the little rod stays under your skin.

The doctor will cover the area with a dressing and a pressure bandage. The pressure bandage will help to stop any bruising and you should leave it on and keep it dry for 24 hours. You should rest your arm for about 12 hours. This means no heavy lifting or exercising during that time. The Implant will settle into your arm and will not be visible, but it can be pushed up to the surface, just under the skin, to be removed.

HOW LONG DOES THE IMPLANT LAST?

Implanon® has been designed to last for three years but you can have it removed whenever you like. After three years, if you want to keep using the Implant as your method of contraception, you can have a new rod inserted when the first one is removed. If you don't want to continue with the Implant and you don't want to be pregnant, you will need to start using another method of contraception right away, because most women find their fertility returns very quickly.

HOW IS THE IMPLANT REMOVED?

Removing the Implant is very simple. You will have another injection of local anaesthetic to make the area feel numb, so it will not hurt. The doctor palpates the Implant, which means they move it using their fingers, up to the surface of your skin. They nick the skin over the end of the Implant with a scalpel and the Implant will slide out with a little pressure. After it is removed, you will have another pressure bandage over the area so it won't develop a large bruise.

Where do I get the Implant?

You need to see a doctor at a Family Planning centre, or a gynaecologist or local doctor who has been trained to insert the Implant. The doctor will give you a prescription that you take to a chemist to get filled. Then you take the Implant back to the doctor to have it inserted.

What does the Implant cost?

Implanon® is on the Pharmaceutical Benefits Scheme (PBS) in Australia and it is available to women with a current Medicare card for about $31. If a woman has a Pharmaceutical Concession Card she will pay much less. If she does not have a Medicare card the Implant will cost about $200. The doctor or Family Planning centre may also charge a fee, in addition to the Medicare fee, to insert the Implant. This fee will vary from doctor to doctor so be sure to ask about this when you are discussing the Implant at the first visit.

Frequently asked questions about implants

Q I know that if you have vomiting or diarrhoea you can lose the effects of the Pill. Is it the same with the Implant?

A No, the Implant will still work to prevent pregnancy because the hormones do not go through your digestive system but are absorbed into your body through your blood stream.

Q I have tried the minipill and DMPA, which I know are also progestogen-only contraceptives. I had problems with both of these. Will that give me any indication of how I will feel with the progestogen-only implant?

A Although these methods all contain only progestogen, they all use different types of progestogen, so they could all have different effects even in the same woman. All progestogens tend to cause irregular bleeding, but it is worth trying others if you have had a problem with one. Even the minipill comes in two types of progestogen, so if one doesn't suit you then the other one might.

Q I am taking the minipill at the moment. Can I just change over to the Implant?

A You can change over quite easily, but you will need to discuss it with your doctor to decide on the best time for you to change.

Q When I have the Implant taken out, will it leave a scar?

A Usually the Implant can be taken out through a very small incision that heals without a noticeable scar. There are some people who will get scarring even with small incisions such as the one used to insert this Implant. If you are unlucky enough to be one of these people, then it is likely the scar will be more obvious when the Implant is removed. The spot chosen to insert the Implant also means that any scar would not be very noticeable.

Q Will it hurt to have the Implant put in?

A No, except for the anaesthetic, which can sting for a few seconds.

Q Will I be able to feel the Implant? Will I know it's there?

A No, you shouldn't be aware of it after the initial discomfort settles down. You usually can't see it but you will feel it if you press down on the skin over the Implant.

Q How quickly will it reverse when I have the Implant removed?

A The effects will be gone in 48 hours. You can expect your periods to return to normal over one to two months.

Things to think about if you are considering the Implant

» You will most likely have unpredictable bleeding from your vagina. This could be either very irregular periods or occasional spotting or bleeding. You could even find that you stop having periods all together.

» There is a slight risk of getting an infection or bleeding at the place on your arm where the Implant is inserted. If it gets red or tender or develops a discharge, you should see a doctor.

» Sometimes women using a progestogen-only implant experience side effects such as headaches or sore breasts. They may put on weight because the progestogen makes them want to eat more. Everyone is different, so you cannot know if you will have any side effects until you have tried the Implant. If you do have unwanted side effects then talk to your doctor to see what you can do.

 HOW TO SAY THESE WORDS

Implanon   *Imp-lan-on*

gynaecologist   *guy-na-coll-a-jist*

palpates   *pal-paits*

7

THE IUD (INTRAUTERINE DEVICE)

The next method I'm going to tell you about is the IUD. IUD stands for intrauterine device, that is, a device that goes inside the uterus. While the IUD is inside the uterus, it prevents pregnancy. There are two types of IUDs available in Australia. You can get a non-hormonal IUD, which does not contain any hormones, or a hormonal IUD. First we'll look at the non-hormonal IUD because it is used more often.

THE NON-HORMONAL IUD

What is a non-hormonal IUD?

The type of non-hormonal IUDs we have in Australia contain copper, and they are generally called copper IUDs, so that's what we will call them now. They are small white plastic devices about 3 centimetres long. They look like a small 'T', or like a small 'T' with the arms curved downwards, with very fine copper wire wrapped around their stems. There is a fine nylon string attached to the end of the stem.

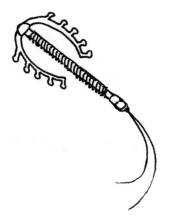

Non-hormonal IUD (copper IUD)

When the IUD is in the uterus, you can feel the string coming through the cervix into the upper end of the vagina. Only about 2 centimetres comes through, so you need to feel right up inside your vagina with your finger to find it. When you can feel the string, you know that the IUD is still in place. The string also makes it easier for a doctor to remove the IUD.

Are there different types of copper IUDs?
There are two different copper IUDs available at present in Australia. They are the Multiload (page 82) and the Copper T.

How does the copper IUD work?
We don't know exactly how it works. We know that it stops sperm from being able to move easily in the uterus and because the sperm cannot swim through the uterus to the tubes to meet an egg, a pregnancy can't begin. Even if a sperm somehow did get to an egg to fertilise it, the action of the IUD touching the lining of the uterus and the copper in the IUD's stem

makes the lining change so a pregnancy cannot grow there.

How effective is the copper IUD?

The copper IUD is more than 98 per cent effective. This means that if 100 women used the copper IUD as their method of contraception for one year, no more than two of them would have an unplanned pregnancy.

Why would I want to choose a copper IUD?

A copper IUD could be a good choice if you have had a baby and you want at least two years between pregnancies. Another reason to choose the copper IUD could be that you have had all the children you want, and you need a very reliable method of contraception, but you would like something that can be reversed easily if you change your mind.

You do not have to remember to use your IUD – it stays in your uterus all the time. You can have an IUD if you are breastfeeding, as it doesn't affect your milk supply. An IUD can protect you against pregnancy for at least five years, and it is relatively inexpensive. Although it costs more than other methods when you first get it, it lasts for a number of years and is good value over time.

Are there any reasons why I could not use a copper IUD?

You should not use an IUD if you are having sex with more than one person, or you have a partner who has sex with other people or you have just started having sex with a new person. This is because if you pick up a sexually transmissible infection from your partner while you are wearing an IUD there is more risk of the infection spreading up to the fallopian tubes and into the abdomen. This sort of infection is known as pelvic inflammatory disease (or PID).

You should not use an IUD if you have had pelvic inflammatory disease more than once in the past or if you could be pregnant. If you have unusual bleeding from your vagina that hasn't been diagnosed, or you have recently had an abnormal Pap test that is being investigated, or you have any signs of genital cancer, then you cannot use an IUD.

Is there anything else that may be a problem if I want to use a copper IUD?

There are some things you should talk over with your doctor if you are considering a copper IUD because these may need to be sorted out before you can have the IUD inserted.

Tell your doctor if you have not had any children but you want to have children in the future. Tell your doctor if your periods are very painful or they last a long time, or both. Periods tend to be heavier and longer when a woman is wearing an IUD, so you may want to think again if your periods are already heavy and long. If you have had an ectopic pregnancy, which is a pregnancy in one of your fallopian tubes, this is also something that needs to be discussed before you have a copper IUD.

If you are anaemic, that is, you don't have enough iron in your blood, or you have fibroids or other conditions that change the shape of your uterus or cervix then you will need to sort these out too. It is also important to consider the risk if you have a medical condition that could affect your recovery if you got an internal infection, for example, if you have rheumatic heart disease, or you are being treated with steroids or other medications that prevent your immune system from working properly.

Where do I get a copper IUD?

To get a copper IUD you need to go to a Family Planning centre, a gynaecologist or a local doctor who has been trained to insert IUDs. You can buy the IUD at most Family Planning centres. A local doctor or gynaecologist may have a supply of IUDs in the surgery or they may give you a prescription to buy the IUD from a chemist before making another appointment to have it inserted.

What does a copper IUD cost?

Both copper IUDs cost about the same. Prices range from about $80 to $100.

WHAT HAPPENS WHEN I HAVE A COPPER IUD INSERTED?

You may be asked to make two medical appointments when you want an IUD. If you have two appointments, the doctor will check to make sure that it is safe for you to have a copper IUD on your first visit. You will be asked questions about your general and reproductive health. Then the doctor will give you an internal examination, which means they will check your vagina and pelvic area. You will also have a Pap test if you are due for one, and possibly tests for vaginal infections.

If you have a second appointment, this is when you will have the IUD inserted. Otherwise, the doctor may insert the IUD at your first appointment, straight after you have been examined. Before the IUD is inserted, you may be given some tablets to relax your muscles or you may have a local anaesthetic, but this is not always needed. In some cases a general anaesthetic may be necessary. Your doctor will tell you what is going to happen.

The procedure takes about 10 minutes. It is not usually painful, though some women find it a bit uncomfortable. You could feel faint while you are having it inserted or soon after. This usually settles quickly. You will be asked to rest for a while, probably about half an hour before you leave the clinic, so the doctor can be sure you are all right.

WHAT SHOULD I EXPECT AFTER A COPPER IUD INSERTION?

You will probably have cramps that are like period cramps, and some bleeding or spotting for a few days after the IUD is inserted. Taking aspirin or paracetemol and holding a hot water bottle or heat pack on your abdomen will help. If you have cramps, spotting or pain for more than a few days, tell your doctor.

You should not have intercourse, that is, penis-in-vagina sex, for three days after the IUD is inserted because of the risk of infection. Nothing should go into your vagina during those three days for the same reason. That means no tampons, baths, swimming or spas for three days. You will need to go back to the doctor for a check-up after six weeks. After that, you can have a check-up when you have your Pap test every two years.

HOW IS THE COPPER IUD REMOVED?

The copper IUD can stay in place from five to ten years, depending on the type. If you want to get pregnant or if you decide that you do not want to have the IUD anymore for other reasons, it can be removed earlier.

You need to see a doctor to have it removed. You will be given another internal examination. Then the doctor will use a special instrument to remove the IUD by gently pulling on the string that comes through the cervix into the vagina. This only takes a couple of minutes. Some women say it feels a bit uncomfortable but some women don't feel much at all.

Things to remember if you use a copper IUD

» If you have an IUD, learn to check the string each month after you have had your period to make sure the IUD is still in the right place.

» If you have any unusual symptoms like a discharge from your vagina or pain low in your belly then you could have an infection, so see your doctor straightaway.

» If your period is more than a week overdue, see your doctor or go to a clinic for a pregnancy test.

» If you or your partner ever have casual sex with another person, of if you have a new sexual partner, use a condom every time you have sex until you both have been checked for sexually transmissible infections (STIs).

Frequently asked questions about copper IUDs

Q Can the man feel the IUD when we have sex?

A The IUD is right inside the uterus so neither you nor your partner can feel it. The man should not even feel the string. If he does and it bothers him, ask your doctor to cut the string shorter.

Q Where does the copper go?

A Every period, a small amount of copper is dissolved in the menstrual blood and comes away with the period. That is why the IUD eventually runs out of copper and you need to get a new IUD.

Things to think about if you are considering a copper IUD

» If you get pregnant while you are using an IUD, there is a slightly higher risk of having an ectopic pregnancy, which is a pregnancy in a fallopian tube. This is still only a very small risk but you should know about it. A pregnancy in a fallopian tube has to be operated on and removed, because there is no room for it to grow and it could be very dangerous for the woman as it can cause internal bleeding.

» There is a greater chance of getting a pelvic infection if you have an IUD. If a woman has a pelvic infection she has more risk of being infertile, which means she may not be able to have children.

» Your periods may be heavier and more painful with a copper IUD and this could be a problem if they are already heavy and painful.

» It is very rare but it is possible that the IUD could be pushed out of the uterus into the vagina and it can even fall out without your noticing. This is more likely to happen during the first few weeks after you've had it inserted, but it can happen at any time. If you don't notice that it has come out, then you're at risk of getting pregnant. This is why you need to check for the string regularly.

» You need to know that, although this is also very rare, it is possible for an IUD to push into the wall of the uterus when it is being inserted, and even more rarely it can go through the wall of the uterus into the abdomen. Remember there is only a tiny chance that this would happen, but if it did, you would need to have an operation to remove it.

» You could become pregnant with the copper IUD in place, although this is also very unlikely. If you find out that you are pregnant and then you have the IUD removed, you have about a 30 per cent chance of miscarriage. If the IUD is not removed, the risk of getting an infection during the pregnancy is higher than normal, and there is also a risk of miscarriage in the last 12 weeks. But most babies will go to full term and can be born normally with an IUD still inside the uterus. The copper IUD does not cause abnormalities in a baby, even when the IUD has been left in place for the whole of the pregnancy because the IUD stays outside the fluid-filled sac where the baby grows.

 ## HOW TO SAY THESE WORDS
Intrauterine *In-tra-you-ter-ine*

THE HORMONAL IUD

What is a hormonal IUD?

A hormonal IUD contains hormones that are chemicals, similar to those that are normally produced in the body to help a woman's reproductive system work properly. The type of hormonal IUD available at present only contains one hormone, progestogen, so we will call it 'the progestogen IUD'. The progestogen IUD is a small white plastic shape about 3 centimetres long, similar to the copper IUD. It looks like a little 'T' (page 90).

The progestogen IUD has a cylinder around the stem with progestogen in it. The cylinder is covered with a membrane that regulates the amount of progestogen released into the uterus. The progestogen IUD also has a fine nylon string attached to the end of the stem. When the IUD is in the uterus, the string comes out through the cervix into the far end of the vagina. If you feel right up inside your vagina with your finger, you can check that the string is there and know it is still in place.

Are there different types of progestogen IUD?

There is only one type of progestogen IUD available in Australia at present. It is called the Mirena®.

How does the progestogen IUD work?

The progestogen IUD affects the lining of the womb so that the lining does not get thick enough for a pregnancy to implant and grow. It makes the mucus in the cervix thicker so that sperm cannot get through to travel up into the uterus. In the first year it is inside the uterus, it also stops ovulation in many women who use it.

How effective is the progestogen IUD?

The progestogen IUD is more than 99 per cent effective. So, if 100 women used the progestogen IUD as their method of contraception for a year, less than one of them would have an unplanned pregnancy. This makes it more effective than the Pill.

Why would I want to choose a progestogen IUD?

Like the copper IUD, the progestogen IUD may be a good choice for you if you have had a baby and you want to have a

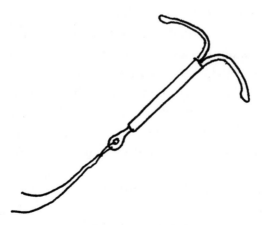

Hormonal IUD (progestogen IUD)

space of two or more years between pregnancies. It could also suit you if you have had all the children you want and you want a very reliable method, but you would also like to know that it can be reversed easily if you change your mind. If you're likely to forget to use contraception, an IUD is a good choice because it is always in place. An IUD is usually easy for most doctors to remove in their surgery.

The thing that is special about the progestogen IUD is that after the first few months you have less menstrual bleeding than with other types of IUD. This is an advantage for women who want an IUD but who normally have heavy periods, or periods that last a long time. And women who get heavy or long-lasting periods if they use a copper IUD can often use a progestogen IUD without any problems.

Are there any reasons why I could not use a progestogen IUD?

Most of the reasons that could prevent you from having a progestogen IUD apply to any IUD and not just those containing progestogen. But because this IUD does contain the hormone progestogen, if you have a medical condition then discuss it with your doctor to make sure it is fine for you to use it. You should not use any IUD if you have sex with more than one person, or your partner has sex with other people, or you have recently started having sex with a new person, because of the risk of infection. This is because you could be at risk of picking up a sexually transmissible infection (STI) from your partner and an IUD inside the uterus increases the risk of that infection spreading up to the fallopian tubes and the abdomen, causing pelvic inflammatory disease (or PID). If you have had PID more than once in the past you should discuss it with your doctor.

If you have bleeding from your vagina that isn't normal

for you and hasn't been diagnosed, or you have signs of genital cancer, you will not be able to have an IUD. If you have
fibroids, or other conditions that change the shape of your
uterus or cervix, you may not be able to have an IUD. If you
could be pregnant then you will need to wait until you are sure
you are not pregnant before having an IUD. While you are
waiting, you should use another method, like condoms, if you
have sex.

Is there anything else that may be a problem if I want to use a progestogen IUD?

There are some things you should talk over with a doctor
so that you can decide how you feel before choosing a progestogen IUD. One issue to discuss is if you have not had a
child but may want to have one in the future. There are some
risks with an IUD that we have talked about already, but it is
best to consider all the possibilities and discuss them with a
doctor before you make a choice.

Some other things that may need to be sorted out include if
you have had an abnormal Pap test that has yet to be treated,
or if you have a medical condition (such as rheumatic heat disease) that makes it very risky for you to get an internal infection. Any condition that means you have to take steroids or
other medications that stop your immune system from working
properly can also be a problem.

If you have already had an IUD and it came out by itself,
tell your doctor. If the space inside your uterus is fairly small
or unusually large, this might mean you are not suitable for an
IUD. The doctor will be able to tell you about this when you
are examined. And if you are going away someplace where you
won't be able to have check-ups after the insertion, it may not
be a good idea to choose a progestogen IUD right now.

Where do I get a progestogen IUD?

You will need to go to a gynaecologist, Family Planning centre or local doctor who has been trained to insert progestogen IUDs. The doctor will give you a prescription to be filled at a chemist and then you take the IUD back to the doctor to have it inserted.

What does a progestogen IUD cost?

The progestogen IUD itself costs about $33 if you have a Medicare card, and is even cheaper with a Health Care Card; otherwise it costs about $240. The doctor may charge an extra fee to insert it. You need to discuss the costs with the doctor before making the appointment to have the IUD inserted.

Although it is more expensive than most other methods when you first buy it, a progestogen IUD can stay in place and protect you against pregnancy for five years. So when you compare it to other methods, the cost is really quite reasonable.

WHAT HAPPENS WHEN I HAVE A PROGESTOGEN IUD INSERTED?

You may be asked to make two appointments if you want a progestogen IUD. The doctor will ask questions about your general and reproductive health on your first visit. You will probably need to have a vaginal/pelvic examination, a Pap test if it is due, and possibly tests for vaginal infections. You will either have the IUD inserted at a second visit, or the doctor will insert it after checking you at the first appointment.

When you are about to have the progestogen IUD inserted, you may be given a muscle relaxant or a local anaesthetic. In some cases a general anaesthetic may be necessary. Your doctor will explain the procedure to you. It takes about 10 minutes and is not usually painful, although some women find it a little uncomfortable. You may feel faint during or after the insertion and you will probably be asked to rest for a while before you leave the clinic so the doctor can be sure you are fine to leave.

WHAT SHOULD I EXPECT AFTER A PROGESTOGEN IUD INSERTION?

You will probably have cramps, like period cramps, and bleeding or spotting during the first few days after the IUD is inserted. If you take aspirin or paracetemol, and hold a hot water bottle or a heat pack on your abdomen, any discomfort you may have will usually settle down. If the cramps last more than a few days, go and see your doctor.

You should not put anything into your vagina for three days after the procedure because of the risk of infection. You should not have vaginal sex, or use tampons, or have baths or spas, or go swimming during that time. You will need to go back to the doctor for a check-up after six weeks. It is quite common for women with a Progestogen IUD to have some spotting or bleeding in the first few months after it is inserted. Once this settles, you just need a check-up every two years with your normal Pap test. At any time, though, if you experience pelvic pain, fever, unusual discharge from your vagina, heavy bleeding, or you think you may be pregnant, you should go to your doctor for another check-up.

HOW IS THE PROGESTOGEN IUD REMOVED?

The progestogen IUD can stay in place for five years. If you want to become pregnant or if you decide that you do not want the IUD anymore for other reasons, it can be removed earlier. You will be given another vaginal/pelvic examination. Then the doctor will use a special instrument to remove the IUD by gently pulling on the string that can be seen coming through the cervix. This only takes a couple of minutes. Some women find it a little uncomfortable but some women don't feel much at all.

Things to remember if you use a progestogen IUD

»   It's really important to learn to check the string each month after a period to make sure your IUD is still in place.

»   If you have any unusual symptoms, like a discharge from your vagina or pain low in your abdomen, you could have an infection, so see your doctor right away.

»   If your period is more than a week overdue, you should see your doctor or go to a clinic for a pregnancy test.

»   If you or your partner ever have casual sex or if you have a new sexual partner, use a condom every time you have sex until you both have been checked for sexually transmissible infections (STIs).

Frequently asked questions about progestogen IUDs

Q   Can a man feel the IUD when we have sex?

A   The IUD is right inside the uterus so neither you nor your partner can feel it. The man should not even feel the string. If he does and it bothers him, ask your doctor to cut the string shorter.

Q   Will I get side effects from the hormones in the progestogen IUD?

A   Most of the hormone stays inside the uterus and works on the lining of the uterus but very small amounts are absorbed into the blood and travel around the body, especially in the first year after the device is inserted. So yes, occasionally women who are very sensitive to progestogens may experience side effects, but these are very rare.

Q   Can I have one of these IUDs if I haven't had any children?

A It is possible to have one of these IUDs inserted if you haven't had any children but they are slightly wider than a copper IUD and may be a little more difficult to put into place.

Q I've heard these might be a good choice for women approaching menopause. Is that right?

A Many women find that as they get into their late forties their periods can become heavier and more irregular. A low dose pill might control this, but the progestogen IUD is another good choice, especially in women who can't or don't want to use the Pill. The progestogen IUD can also be left inside up to its five-year life span to provide one of the hormones given in hormone replacement therapy (HRT).

Things to think about if you are considering a progestogen IUD

» Your periods will change and you are likely to have irregular bleeding for the first three to five months after you have a progestogen IUD inserted. If you keep the IUD for longer than this, it is common to have very few periods.

» In rare cases, the IUD could be pushed out of the uterus into the vagina and can even fall out, perhaps when you go to the toilet. If you don't notice that this has happened, you will be at risk of getting pregnant. That is why you need to check for the string regularly. However, if the IUD is going to come out, it is more likely to do so during the first few weeks after it has been inserted. The chance of the progestogen IUD coming out by itself is slightly higher than with a copper IUD.

» The risk of ectopic pregnancy (pregnancy in a fallopian tube) is *very* low with a progestogen IUD.

» There is more chance of getting a pelvic infection with any type of IUD. If a woman has a pelvic infection, she has increased risk of infertility, which means she may not be able to have children.

» Very rarely, during insertion, the IUD can pass into the wall of the uterus, and even more rarely through the wall of the uterus into the abdominal cavity. If this did happen, you would need to have an operation to remove it.

» Very occasionally, a woman becomes pregnant with the Progestogen IUD in place. If the IUD is removed, there is about a 30 per cent chance that the woman will have a miscarriage. There are possible complications in continuing a pregnancy if the progestogen IUD is not removed straightaway.

» There is a slight chance that there may be other side effects with the progestogen IUD. Approximately three per cent of women using the progestogen IUD have symptoms such as dry vagina, flushing, headaches, nausea, acne, and mood changes. If you experience any of these symptoms, talk to your doctor to see what can be done to help relieve them.

HOW TO SAY THESE WORDS

Mirena® *Me-ray-na*

rheumatic *roo-mat-ick*

8

NATURAL METHODS

BASIC FACTS ABOUT NATURAL FAMILY PLANNING

What is natural family planning?

Natural family planning, or NFP, is based on the idea that if you understand your own menstrual cycle then you can predict the times when you are most likely to be fertile. It is called natural family planning because you do not use any artificial devices or chemical hormones. You just pay attention to the natural changes in your body and only have sex when you feel that all the signs tell you that you are very unlikely to become pregnant.

You may hear natural methods called fertility awareness methods, or FAM. Being fertile means that you are quite likely to become pregnant if you have sex without using any contraception. Most women are fertile for up to eight days of each menstrual cycle. This may surprise you, because generally we think that women only get pregnant when they ovulate, but although the egg only lives for about 24 hours, sperm can live for several days inside a woman's uterus and fallopian tubes. In fact, it is possible for sperm to survive there for up to seven days, and if that happened, you just might become pregnant even if you had not had sex for nearly a week before you ovulated.

If you do not have vaginal sex during your fertile time, there won't be any sperm in your body to meet the egg and fertilise it.

Are there different types of natural family planning?

There are four ways to work out when you are likely to be fertile. These are the calendar method, the temperature method, the Billings (mucus) method and a combination of these that is usually known as the sympto-thermal method.

For now, I will give you a brief description of each one, but if you decide to try a natural method it is important to see a natural family planning specialist. A person who knows the details of the method can tell you all the physical signs and symptoms to watch for, so that you have the best possible chance to use the method effectively.

What is the calendar method?

The calendar method is sometimes called the rhythm method. It is based on the fact that most women ovulate between 12 and 16 days before a period begins. You use the calendar to work out when your period is likely to come, and then you can work out when you are likely to ovulate. If you do not have sex at that time, you can avoid becoming pregnant.

HOW DO I USE THE CALENDAR METHOD?

You will need to write down the length of each menstrual cycle for six months or however long it takes you to have six cycles. A menstrual cycle is measured by counting the first day of a period as day one. The next day is day two. You keep on counting like this even when your period finishes. Count each day until your next period starts. That is one cycle. Write down the number of days in that cycle. When the next period starts, you start at day one again and count the days of that next cycle.

An average menstrual cycle is about 28 days, but your cycle may be only 21 days or it could be as long as 35 days (or even longer). This is usually nothing to be worried about – you just need to know what is normal for you. Some women will find they have cycles of different lengths from month to month. Most women will need some help from a natural family planning specialist to work out their fertile days if they want to use this method effectively, but here's a guide to how it's done.

If you have sex, during the time that you are recording the length of your cycles, you should use another method of contraception like condoms, or avoid having vaginal sex. You should definitely not be using the Pill or the minipill, the vaginal ring, the contraceptive injection, the contraceptive implant, or the hormonal IUD, because you do not have normal cycles while you are using a hormonal method of contraception.

At the end of six cycles you can calculate your fertile time. Write down the length of the shortest cycle. Let's say it was 26 days. Now take away 20 from that number, in this case we've said it is 26, and that leaves 6.

Then write down the length of your longest cycle. Let's say that was 30 days. Take away 10 from that number, and we have 20. Look at the two numbers, 6 and 20. They mean that your unsafe days are from day 6 to day 20 of your cycle. So, sometime between the sixth day after your period starts and the twentieth day after your period starts, you might be ovulating and so it is not safe for you to have unprotected sex during that time.

Of course, you will not be fertile all that time, but you cannot be sure exactly when you are going to ovulate, so this covers you for most possibilities. Some other systems use slightly different numbers, and that is why it is best to go and see someone who has taught the method a lot, and can explain it to you properly.

What is the Billings (mucus) method?

During your menstrual cycle your cervix produces mucus that changes from dry to wet and stringy, and then back to dry again. When you know what these changes mean, you can tell when you are likely to be fertile, and can avoid having sex at that time.

HOW DO I USE THE BILLINGS (MUCUS) METHOD?

The mucus method relies on you noticing changes in the mucus at the opening of your vagina every morning when you wake up. You feel just inside the vaginal opening with your finger and notice if you feel wet or dry. If there is any mucus on your finger you can see what it looks like. Depending on what the mucus looks and feels like, you can tell whether you are fertile or not. Then you know whether it is safe to have sex that day.

There are three different types of mucus to check for. As soon as your period finishes, your vaginal opening will feel dry, and any mucus will be thick, flaky and sticky. Around the time that you are ovulating, your vagina will feel wet, and the mucus will be clear, watery and stretchy, like egg white. After you ovulate, the mucus will be cloudy, thicker, and sticky again, and your vagina will feel dry around the opening. With this method you can presume you are safe three days after you last feel the slippery wet mucus.

There are several things you must do to use this method as safely as possible. Firstly, in the early part of your cycle before ovulation, you can only have intercourse every second day because if there is any semen from the man in your vagina you would not be able to tell if there is any mucus there. Secondly, you can only have intercourse on a day when you have felt dry in the morning. Thirdly, if you have any bleeding or spotting during the cycle, you must treat that the same as fertile mucus.

What is the temperature method?

The temperature method is based on the fact that when you ovulate, your body temperature rises between 0.2 and 0.5 degrees Celsius and it stays that way until your next period starts, then it drops down again. The next period usually starts between 12 and 16 days after you ovulate.

HOW DO I USE THE TEMPERATURE METHOD?

You have to take your temperature every day to find out when you ovulate so that you can work out your safe time. You must take your temperature every morning as soon as you wake up, before you get out of bed. It also has to be taken before you eat, drink or smoke.

This is called your basal body temperature (bbt). Your basal body temperature is your temperature when your body is completely at rest.

You can take your temperature with the thermometer in your mouth or in your vagina, but you will need to decide on one or the other and do that for the whole cycle. Be aware that your temperature can go up for a number of reasons, like illness, for example. It should be safe to have sex once you have had three days, one after the other, where the readings are higher than on any of the six days before them.

I'll say that another way. Take your temperature every day from the first day of a period, and record the temperature on a chart or graph. You will see that for a number of days your temperature will stay just about the same, then one day you should notice that the temperature has gone up a bit. If it is still up on the following day, and then the day after that (three days), and it is higher on each of those three days than on any of the six days before it went up, that means you have ovulated. It also means your fertile time is now over and it is safe to have unprotected sex.

You will notice that this method only gives you a safe period in the second half of the cycle *after* you have ovulated and isn't able to give you any idea of your fertile times early in the cycle. This means that if you use this method correctly and have a 28-day cycle, there are probably only 11 days a month when this method says you are safe from pregnancy.

What is the sympto-thermal method?

The sympto-thermal method combines the calendar, temperature, and mucus methods. You use aspects of all of them to work out when you are fertile and when it is safe for you to have unprotected sex. A natural family planning specialist is the best person to explain this method to you.

How effective is natural family planning?

It is difficult to be accurate about the effectiveness of natural methods. We know that natural methods become more effective the longer they are practised. They are also more effective if people are very motivated to use them. Some natural family planning specialists believe that if you use a natural method exactly as you are instructed, it can be up to 98 per cent effective. The problem is that because people forget or make mistakes with their calculations or for all sorts of other reasons they do not use the method as instructed, it is often much less reliable.

So if you think about it, you will see that you have to be absolutely committed to using this type of method correctly for it to work for you. Some people combine a natural method with the use of a barrier method, like condoms, when they think the woman could be fertile. Then of course it's important that you use the condom correctly too.

Why would I want to choose natural family planning?

You may want to choose a natural method of contraception if you prefer a method that does not involve using any device, and does not affect your whole system. You may want to use a natural method if you have religious beliefs that prevent you from using artificial contraception, especially if natural methods are acceptable to you.

If you are intending to have a baby in the not-too-distant future, or if an unexpected pregnancy would not be a problem, you might like to have a rest from other methods and rely on a natural method. Natural methods are free after the initial cost of consultations and possibly the cost of a thermometer and charts. You may like to choose a natural method because both partners share the responsibility for contraception, and some couples find that this is very good for their relationship.

Are there any reasons why I could not use natural family planning?

If your partner is not prepared to cooperate, or could be unreliable, you probably won't be able to use a natural method. If you are not prepared to take note of your physical changes every day, or you are not prepared to avoid vaginal sex for fairly long periods of time, then a natural method would not be a good choice.

If an unplanned pregnancy would cause serious problems,

then you would not be advised to use a natural method unless there really is no other choice, because the risk of failure would be too great.

Frequently asked questions about natural family planning

Q I've heard there are personal fertility tests and even a fertility computer that can make the calculations of fertile days easier. Are these available in Australia?

A There are several products that you can buy at a chemist that you can use to see if you are ovulating. There is a little hand-held computer with the trade name Persona® that analyses homones in a woman's urine and gradually builds up a pattern of her fertile and non-fertile times. Check with your local chemist, but if it is not available it may be possible to order one online from Britain where they are made and are used by many women choosing natural family planning methods.

Q Can I successfully use natural family planning as I get older and my natural fertility decreases anyway?

A Anyone can learn to recognise the changes in their body that signal the beginning of a fertile time in the cycle. As you get older, though, the cycles tend to be a bit more irregular and it can become a little more difficult to rely on your previous cycle length.

Q Can I use this method to help me get pregnant if I want to?

A Yes the very same changes can be used to help a woman predict the most fertile time in her cycle and therefore increase her chances of becoming pregnant if that is what she wants to do.

Things to think about if you are considering using natural family planning

» If you are worried that you have made a mistake in your calculations, and you have had sex when you are probably fertile, you have the choice to use the emergency contraceptive pill. But be aware that if you use it, your menstrual cycle will most likely change over the next month or so, and you will not be able to rely on a natural method until your cycles return to what is normal for you.

» Remember that both partners have to be committed to using a natural method for it to be effective.

» Natural methods do not give you any protection against sexually transmissible infections (STIs).

HOW TO SAY THESE WORDS

basal *bay-sal*

Persona *Per-sone-a*

Sympto-thermal *sim-toe-ther-mal*

9

TRADITIONAL METHODS

When we talk about traditional methods of contraception, we mean methods that have been used by people of many different cultures for many generations. The two traditional methods we will look at are breastfeeding and the withdrawal method. First, let's talk about breastfeeding.

BREASTFEEDING

Why is breastfeeding called a method of contraception?

Most women do not have periods while they are fully breast-feeding their babies. Fully breastfeeding means that you are not giving the baby any other foods, or bottles of milk or formula. Because they are not having periods, many women think they cannot become pregnant, so they use breastfeeding as their method of contraception. We now know that it is possible for breastfeeding women to become pregnant even if they have not had a period since their baby was born, but we will talk about that a bit later.

How does breastfeeding stop me becoming pregnant?

When a baby sucks on the breast, the mother's body has a hormonal response. This hormonal response affects the mother's ovaries and stops them from releasing any eggs. If there is no egg available to be fertilised then there will be no pregnancy.

How effective is breastfeeding as a method of contraception?

Breastfeeding can be 98 per cent effective if each of the following three conditions apply to you: Firstly, you are not having periods. Secondly, you are fully breastfeeding your baby. Remember, fully breastfeeding means that you are not giving the baby any other foods, or bottles of milk or formula. Thirdly, it is no more than six months since your baby was born.

If 100 women used breastfeeding as their method of contraception for six months, and all those conditions applied to them, probably only two of them would have an unplanned pregnancy during that time.

By the time the baby is 12 months old, the effectiveness of breastfeeding in preventing pregnancy will have reduced to 93 per cent. This means that if 100 women used breastfeeding as their method of contraception during that year, by the end of twelve months seven of them would have had an unplanned pregnancy. This would happen even if they had not had a period since their baby was born and they were still fully breastfeeding.

Why would I want to choose breastfeeding as a method of contraception?

If you want to fully breastfeed your baby and you are prepared to accept a slight risk of another pregnancy during the first six months, then it may suit you just to rely on breastfeeding.

It may especially suit you if you intend to have another child eventually, and would be able to accept an unexpected pregnancy were it to happen. Other reasons for choosing to rely on breastfeeding for a while are that it is free, and it gives you the opportunity to have a rest from using other methods of contraception.

Are there any reasons why I could not use breastfeeding as a method of contraception?

If you do not produce enough milk to fully breastfeed, you would not be able to rely on breastfeeding to protect you against pregnancy. If you have HIV, you would not be advised to breastfeed because the virus can pass on to the baby through your milk. If you are working, you may not be able to breastfeed frequently enough to keep up the level of hormones your body needs to prevent ovulation.

HOW DO I USE BREASTFEEDING FOR CONTRACEPTION?

Well, the three things we discussed earlier – no periods, fully breastfeeding, and your baby under six months old – are very important. The main thing for you to do then is to make sure that your baby sucks frequently.

Sucking on the nipple causes your uterus to contract and also causes your body to release a hormone called prolactin, which helps in the production of breast milk. Prolactin can also prevent ovulation.

Frequently asked questions about breastfeeding to prevent pregnancy

Q If you're not having any periods, how can you get pregnant?

A The first period comes about two weeks after the first ovulation, so it is possible to get pregnant even before you know your body has started to have regular periods again. Also, if you're not used to having regular periods then it might be several months before you even realise that you could be pregnant.

Q I got some light bleeding for a couple of months after I had my last baby. Does this count as a period if I want to use breastfeeding for contraception?

A This light bleeding is called lochia and is it is quite normal to get this, usually on and off, for up to six weeks after having a baby. As long as it is light, and as long as it is less than two months since you had the baby, it doesn't count as a period. Heavy period-like bleeding (even early on), or light bleeding later than two months, probably does count as a period, and you should see your doctor or Family Planning centre for advice.

Things to think about if you are considering using breastfeeding as your contraception

» After your baby is born, you will ovulate before you have your first period.

» If you are fully breastfeeding, you may not have a period until you start giving the baby extra bottles of milk or formula, or solid food. You may not have a period until you stop breastfeeding altogether. On the other hand, be aware that your periods can start at any time. Everyone is different.

» It is a good idea to start using some other method as well as breastfeeding, from six months after the baby is born. Barrier methods, the minipill, a progestogen-only implant or an IUD are all good methods to think about because none of them will affect your ability to continue breastfeeding. In most cases the combined pill can be used while you are breastfeeding after the baby is six months old.

» Even if you decide not to rely on breastfeeding for contraception, remember that breastfeeding is good for babies. It is also a convenient feeding method if you have enough milk for your baby and you can organise your life so that you can be available to breastfeed. Breast milk provides a good balance of nutrients for young babies and it gives them greater protection from infection than formula or cow's milk.

 HOW TO SAY THESE WORDS

lochia *lock-ee-ya*

prolactin *pro-lack-tin*

WITHDRAWAL

Another traditional method is called the withdrawal method. It is usually just called 'withdrawal', so that's what we will call it. It is also known as coitus interruptus, or 'being careful'. Withdrawal is not talked about much or recommended anymore, as there are so many other reliable methods available, but it has been used fairly successfully for centuries.

What is withdrawal?

Withdrawal involves the man removing his penis from the woman's vagina just before he ejaculates or 'comes'.

How does withdrawal work?

If the man does not come inside the woman, there will be no sperm in the fallopian tubes to meet an egg and start a pregnancy.

How effective is withdrawal?

Withdrawal has not been studied a lot as a method of contraception, but it is thought to be quite effective as long as the couple is committed to using it and the man has enough control to do it properly.

HOW DO I USE WITHDRAWAL?

You have sex until the man feels that he is about to come. Then he pulls out of the woman's vagina and ejaculates somewhere away from the entrance to her vagina, so that semen does not get inside her.

Why would I want to choose withdrawal?

You may want to choose withdrawal if a situation arises where you have sex unexpectedly and there is no other method available. You may want to use it as a backup to another method, particularly a natural method. Some people choose withdrawal so they can have a rest from other methods, especially when an unexpected pregnancy would not be a problem. Withdrawal doesn't cost anything and is always available.

Is there any reason why I could not use withdrawal?

Withdrawal depends a lot on the man's control over his ejaculation. If he experiences premature ejaculation, which means he comes very quickly and can't help it, you would not be able to use this method unless he is able to learn a technique that gives him more control. Contact a Family Planning centre or your local doctor to find out about this technique.

Frequently asked questions about withdrawal

Q I have heard that there is sperm in the pre-cum on the tip of a man's penis before he ejaculates. Can't I get pregnant from that?

A There may be a few sperm in this fluid and while it is possible to get pregnant with only very small numbers of sperm it is also very unlikely. Most pregnancies that occur when a couple are using withdrawal happen because the man pulls out too late and large numbers of sperm are left near the entrance to the vagina.

Things to think about if you are considering using withdrawal

» Some people find the sudden ending to intercourse is very frustrating and some women feel unsatisfied if they have not had an orgasm before the man withdraws, so if this happens regularly it may become a problem. On the other hand it does not bother some people at all.

» Both partners must be committed to using withdrawal and feel happy about it, for it to be successful.

HOW TO SAY THESE WORDS

Coitus *coy-tiss*

Interruptus *in-ter-up-tiss*

10

EMERGENCY CONTRACEPTION

As its name implies, emergency contraception is meant to be used in an emergency. It is something that is designed to prevent you from becoming pregnant if you have sex and then realise that you were not protected.

We've already talked about using emergency contraception if your usual method fails. If your condom breaks or slips off, or if you completely forget to use contraception, you may want to use emergency contraception. No matter how it happens, you have the choice to use emergency contraception, but you need to use it fairly quickly. It is more effective the sooner it is used after you have had unprotected sex, and it must be used within five days.

When we talk about emergency contraception we usually mean the emergency contraceptive pill. Having a copper IUD inserted is also considered to be a method of emergency contraception, although it is very rarely used in Australia. I will tell you about the emergency contraceptive pill first.

THE EMERGENCY CONTRACEPTIVE PILL (ECP)

What is the emergency contraceptive pill?

The emergency contraceptive pill used to be called 'the morning-after pill'. You may hear it referred to as ECP, or post-coital contraception. The emergency contraceptive pill is really just a special dose of the hormones used in oral contraceptive pills.

Are there different types of emergency contraceptive pills?

There are two types of emergency contraceptive pill. One method is a special dose of the hormone progestogen that you take as either a single pill, or as two pills. The other method, which doctors call the Yuzpe method, uses combined oral contraceptive pills, but this method is not used much any more.

How do emergency contraceptive pills work?

If you take emergency pills before you have ovulated, they will stop or delay an egg being released that month. If you take them after you have ovulated, they can cause changes in the lining of the uterus that will stop a fertilised egg from implanting and growing there.

How effective is the emergency contraceptive pill?

It is not easy to know exactly how effective emergency contraceptive pills are, but it is thought that the progestogen-only method is about 85 per cent effective and the combined method is about 74 per cent effective.

Why would I want to use emergency contraception?

You may want to use emergency contraception if you have sex and then realise you were not protected against pregnancy, and you absolutely do not want to be pregnant. Some women may only want to use it if they had sex around the time that they would expect to be ovulating. If a woman is sexually assaulted she may want to use emergency contraception.

Are there any reasons why I could not use the emergency contraceptive pill?

There is no medical reason that would stop you using the progestogen-only method, except if you are pregnant already. Even then, emergency contraception will not affect the pregnancy – it just won't work if the foetus has already implanted in the uterus.

Some doctors would not recommend that you use the combined pill method if you have had blood clots in your legs or lungs or if you suffer from a severe kind of migraine called focal migraine. Some women have severe nausea when they take this amount of oestrogen, so the progestogen-only method could be a better option for them.

Where do I get the emergency contraceptive pill?

You can buy the one- or two-pack emergency contraceptive pills at a chemist without a doctor's prescription. The chemist may ask you some questions about your health to make sure it is safe for you to take it.

You need to go to a doctor for a prescription for the combined emergency contraceptive pills, but this method should only be used if the one- or two-pack emergency pills are not available.

What do emergency contraception pills cost?

The progestogen-only pill method of emergency contraception costs about $30 from the chemist and a little less from Family Planning centres.

HOW DO I USE THE EMERGENCY CONTRACEPTIVE PILL?

Now there is a one-pack emergency pill that is very simple to use. It is just a single pill containing a type of progestogen (levonorgestrel 1.5 milligrams). Its trade name is Postinor-1®. You need to take this pill as soon as possible, and no longer than 120 hours (five days) after unprotected sex.

There are several two-pack emergency pills available, which use the same type of progestogen as Postinor-1® but with half the dose (0.75mg) in each pill. Their trade names are Postinor-2®, Levonelle-2®, or NorLevo®. These packs have two pills: you take one pill as soon as possible after unprotected sex, and the other pill exactly 12 hours later.

Women don't usually feel sick with the progestogen-only method. Some women get sore breasts and some have irregular periods for a while after taking it.

The combined pill method is an older kind of emergency contraception, using pills containing the two hormones oestrogen and progestogen. It involves taking one dose of pills (two or four pills, depending on the type of pill used) as soon as possible after unprotected sex. Then you take another dose, exactly 12 hours later. The doctor will tell you which type of pill you have been given and how many to take.

Some women have quite severe nausea with the combined pill method, although it usually does not last more than 12 hours after the second dose of pills. If you use this method, ask the doctor for anti-nausea pills to take with each dose. Some women get sore breasts or changes to their periods with shorter or longer cycles for a while after they have taken this method of emergency contraception.

Frequently asked questions about the emergency contraceptive pill

Q If I take the pills and they don't work and I get pregnant, will they affect the baby?

A No, the hormones in these emergency pills do not cause birth defects.

Q Should I get the emergency contraceptive pill if I miss a couple of days of my normal contraceptive pill?

A You may be advised to take the emergency contraceptive pill if you miss two or more hormone pills at the beginning or end of your Pill pack, that is, just before or just after the pill-free or dummy pill week. You would probably need to miss quite a few pills in the middle of your Pill packet before emergency contraception would be advisable. If you feel worried or unsure what to do, ring a Family Planning centre or talk to your doctor.

Q Do I need a check-up after I've taken emergency contraception?

A You only need to have a check-up if your period is more then a week late, or the bleeding is lighter then usual, or you have spotting, or sex is painful.

Things to think about if you are considering the emergency contraceptive pill

» The emergency contraceptive pill works best if it is used within 24 hours after unprotected sex. It becomes less effective as time passes, but it must be taken within five days.

» It may be that you need to use a more reliable method of contraception. Talk to your doctor to help you decide what to do.

HOW TO SAY THESE WORDS

levonorgestrel *lev-owe-nor-jess-trel*

Yuzpe *Yuzz-pea*

AN IUD IN AN EMERGENCY

I mentioned in the previous session that, although it is very rarely used, there is the alternative of having an IUD inserted for emergency contraception.

How does the IUD work as emergency contraception?

If you have an IUD inserted, it causes changes in the lining of the uterus. If an egg is fertilised and makes its way to the uterus it cannot implant in the lining and grow there.

How effective is it?

Insertion of a copper IUD within five days of unprotected sex is more than 99 per cent effective at preventing pregnancy. It has to be a copper IUD to be effective, because hormonal IUDs take too long to work to be useful for emergency contraception.

HOW DO I USE THE IUD FOR EMERGENCY CONTRACEPTION?

You just have the IUD inserted no more than five days after you have had unprotected sex. See chapter 7 for information about a copper IUD, and where to get it. The only difference is that in this case you have an IUD inserted because you think you are at risk of becoming pregnant and you want to reduce that risk. You can, of course, choose to have the IUD removed after the next period, though few people actually decide to do this having gone to the trouble and expense of having the IUD inserted in the first place.

What does it cost?

A copper IUD costs from between $80 and $100 and can be bought at a chemist or a Family Planning centre. You may also need to pay some medical costs for the doctor to insert the device so check the costs before deciding to go ahead with the insertion.

Things to think about if you are considering an IUD for emergency contraception

» Do you need to use more reliable contraception? If you think you do, the copper IUD may be a good idea if it is suitable for you, because it will act as emergency contraception and then stay in place for up to ten years.

11

STERILISATION

FEMALE STERILISATION (TUBAL LIGATION)

Sterilisation is a permanent method of contraception. Sterilisation for a woman means that she has an operation to close off her fallopian tubes and then she cannot have children anymore. Female sterilisation is often called tubal ligation, which means 'tying the tubes', so from now on we will call it tubal ligation. There is a new method of blocking the fallopian tubes by placing micro-inserts in the tubes. We will discuss this in the next session.

Some women have a hysterectomy, which is the removal of the uterus, when they decide on sterilisation. You can discuss hysterectomy with your doctor if you wish, but it is not necessary to have such a big operation just to stop you falling pregnant. A hysterectomy would normally only be done if you have some other medical problem with your uterus.

What is tubal ligation?

Tubal ligation involves a woman having an operation to block her fallopian tubes in some way (page 123). It is done under either a local or a general anaesthetic.

Are there different types of tubal ligation?

The most common method of tubal ligation is done by using Filshie clips, one on each tube. Filshie clips are made of titanium, which is a type of metal, lined with silicone rubber. They have a tight locking device that does not leave any space for an egg to pass through when it clamps the walls of the fallopian tube together. They are made in a special curved shape

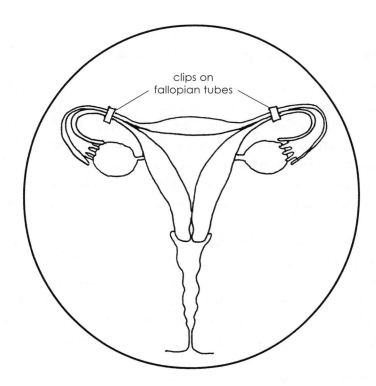

clips on
fallopian tubes

Female sterilisation (tubal ligation with clips)

that makes them very easy for a doctor to put in place.

There are a number of other ways to block a woman's fallopian tubes, including:

» electrocautery, where an electric current is applied to each tube, creating a blockage by making the walls stick together
» fallope rings, which are bands made of silastic (a type of plastic). They close off the tubes and over time the parts of the tubes that are squeezed closed harden and become permanently blocked.
» Hulka clips, which are spring-loaded plastic clips that work in a similar way to Filshie clips
» removal of part of the tubes, when the tubes are blocked or tied in two places and the portion between is cut and removed. This takes a longer operation and a longer stay in hospital.
» a relatively new method of female sterilisation using micro-inserts, which we will talk about next.

How does tubal ligation work?

Whatever method is used, tubal ligation stops the egg from going all the way along the fallopian tube to meet the sperm and it stops the sperm from travelling up the fallopian tube to meet the egg.

How effective is tubal ligation?

Tubal ligation is very effective. Some methods are slightly more effective than others. If one thousand women (that's 1000, not 100 women) had Filshie clips as their method of tubal ligation, after one year, only two or three of them would have an unexpected pregnancy. If they had another method, possibly up to nine women out of 1000 would have become pregnant. Unfortunately, these failure rates are for the first year only and it is believed that the failure rates of many of these methods will increase as time passes from the operation. So that if we talk about lifetime failure rates, the real figure might be that 1 in 200 women finds that she is pregnant after a tubal ligation has been performed and one-third of those pregnancies will be ectopic or tubal pregnancies, which can be quite dangerous, and would require an operation to remove them.

Why would I want to choose tubal ligation?
You may want to choose tubal ligation if you have children and feel you do not want any more. You may want to choose tubal ligation if do not have any children but are sure you do not ever want to have them. You may also decide on a tubal ligation if you have a condition that would make it dangerous for you to be pregnant or give birth, or if you have a genetic disorder that may be passed on to your child if you had one.

Are there any reasons why I could not have a tubal ligation?
There are no reasons that would absolutely prevent you from having a tubal ligation. But sometimes the risk of having a tubal ligation has to be weighed against the risk of pregnancy.

Are there any other things that could cause problems with a tubal ligation?
You may not be able to have a tubal ligation if you have had a pelvic infection recently or if you have any illness that could cause problems with the anaesthetic or surgery. You will most likely be advised not to have a tubal ligation at the same time as an abortion. Tubal ligation is not usually recommended just after having a baby because the failure rate is higher if it is done then. In fact, it is usually suggested that you wait to have a tubal ligation until your baby is over 12 months old, since

very young babies are the ones most at risk of cot death. If you are very overweight, you will not be able to have a laparoscopy, which is one of the most common ways that tubal ligation is done.

HOW IS A TUBAL LIGATION DONE?

Tubal ligation is most often done by laparoscopy. A laparoscope is like a little telescope that can be used inside the pelvis. It has a fibre optic light that allows the doctor to see exactly where your tubes are. It is inserted into the abdomen through a small incision about 1 centimetre long, just under your belly button. The abdomen is filled with carbon dioxide gas so that the organs separate and can be easily seen and accessed. You will probably have another small incision near your pubic hairline, just above your pubic bone, so that the instrument that does the sterilisation procedure can be inserted through there.

There is another procedure called a mini laparotomy, which involves having a slightly larger incision near the pubic hairline. Another kind of instrument that helps the doctor to see inside easily is inserted through the incision in your abdomen. A second instrument is inserted through your vagina into the uterus and pushes the uterus and tubes into a position where the doctor can work with them. Both laparoscopy and mini laparotomy can be done with a local anaesthetic, but are more commonly done in Australia under general anaesthetic.

Some women have a laparotomy. With this method you will need to have a general anaesthetic and you will stay in hospital for a few days. You will have a larger incision, about 7 centimetres long, across the lower part of your abdomen. Each fallopian tube is lifted up and tied or clipped. Sometimes the doctor will remove a part of the tube between two ties.

WHAT CAN I EXPECT AFTER A TUBAL LIGATION?

Some women can feel a bit sick in the stomach for a few days after any general anaesthetic. After tubal ligation most women will feel some crampy discomfort in their lower abdomen and maybe some pain or skin irritation where the stitches are. This would usually last for two to five days after the operation. Women who have had a laparoscopy can also expect some pain in their shoulder tip. This is because the gas used to inflate the abdomen before the operation may cause irritation to the nerves that supply a small area of skin at the shoulder tip.

Medication from the chemist, such as paracetamol, will usually help, but if the pain gets worse or the paracetamol doesn't help, you really need to contact your doctor for advice.

Where do I have tubal ligation surgery?

You need to go to a hospital or day surgery to have a tubal ligation. First you must see your local doctor or a doctor at a Family Planning centre to talk about it and get a referral to the specialist who actually does the surgery. The specialist will help you arrange things from there, including where you can go to have the surgery, how much it will cost, and so on.

What does a tubal ligation cost?

The cost varies according to the method used, and how long you have to stay in hospital. If you are not in a health insurance fund, but you are covered by Medicare and go to a public hospital for day surgery, it may not cost you anything but there could be quite a long wait to have it done. Be sure to sort out the costs you will face with the doctor who will be performing the operation before you book in for surgery, and to check first with your health insurance fund if you are thinking of making a claim through them.

Frequently asked questions about tubal ligation

Q Does my partner have to give consent or sign anything if I want to have a tubal ligation?

A No, you don't need your partner's consent. Of course it is good to talk over such a big decision together and it is best if you agree, but in the end it is your body and your decision.

Q Even though I know the chance is very small, I've heard that you might still get pregnant after you've had a tubal ligation. How can that happen?

A It is possible for the tubes to somehow join up again or at least get close enough so that an egg and sperm can meet even many years after the operation. Sometimes, if this happens, the pregnancy grows in a fallopian tube instead of the uterus. This is called an ectopic pregnancy, and it has to be removed because there is no room for it to grow. If it were left there it would be very dangerous for the woman as it can cause internal bleeding.

Q If I have a tubal ligation, will that bring on menopause?

A No, tubal ligation has no effect on menopause. Your ovaries function as usual and you still have periods until you would normally experience menopause.

Q Will the tubal ligation affect the way I feel about sex?

A No. Other than being relieved that you are free from the risk of pregnancy, you should not notice any other changes to the way you feel about sex. Tubal ligation has no physical effect on your body other than to block the egg from meeting a sperm and being fertilised.

Q I have heard that tubal ligation is reversible – that you can have an operation to join the tubes and you can get pregnant again. Is this true?

A It is true that most people (though not everyone) can have an operation to rejoin the tubes but, even after this, many people still don't become pregnant. We don't really know why. The scar tissue could make it difficult for eggs and sperm to get past. There are several ideas about it, but the main thing is that there is no guarantee that a reversal of a tubal ligation will work. Some women these days are having in-vitro fertilisation (IVF) rather than having surgery done to unblock the tubes, but again the success rate is not all that high.

You should see the decision to have a tubal ligation as a final one. So if you have any doubts about having this procedure, it is best to wait and use another method of contraception until you feel sure it is what you want. And if your life changes later on in ways you had not thought of, and you regret having the tubal ligation, you will at least know that you had considered everything carefully and felt it really was the best decision at the time.

Things to think about if you are considering tubal ligation

» It is usually best to have a tubal ligation separate from other big events in your life, especially if they are stressful. You are more likely to regret having a tubal ligation if it is done when you have an abortion, or straight after you have a baby, or if you are having problems with your relationship.

» If you have a tubal ligation for medical reasons, rather than because you chose to have it, you may have a lot of mixed feelings about it. You could find that talking to a counsellor or a trusted friend or family member will help.

» Remember that tubal ligation is an operation and, like all operations, there is a risk of complications. If you are generally healthy, the risk with this procedure is very small.

» Only choose sterilisation after thinking it over very carefully. If you already have children, you need to feel as sure as possible that no matter what happens in your life you would not want to have another child. If you have never had children, then it may be an even bigger decision to make.

» Sterilisation does not protect you from sexually transmissible infections (STIs), so you may want to use condoms as well.

 HOW TO SAY THESE WORDS

Filshie *fill-she*
hysterectomy *his-ter-eck-toe-me*
laparoscopy *lap-are-oss-cop-ee*
laparotomy *lap-are-otto-me*
silastic *sye-lass-tick*
tubal ligation *tube-al lie-gay-shun*

FEMALE STERILISATION (MICRO-INSERTS)

In this session we are looking at another method of blocking the fallopian tubes using 'micro-inserts'. I have made it a separate session because the procedure is quite different to tubal ligation and does not involve cutting through your skin to access the fallopian tubes.

What are micro-inserts?

Micro-inserts are very small, flexible devices that are placed inside the fallopian tubes to prevent pregnancy (see illustration below).

Are there different types of micro-inserts?

There is only one type of micro-insert available at present. It is called the Essure® procedure. The Essure® procedure has micro-inserts that look like little spirals. These are made of a material that has been used in heart surgery and other surgical procedures for a long time.

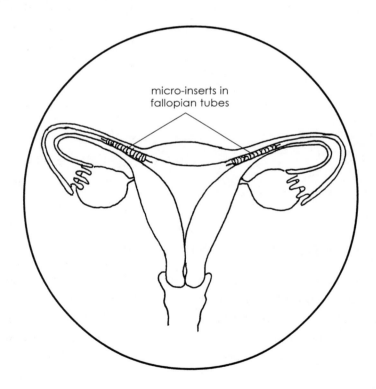

micro-inserts in
fallopian tubes

Female sterilisation (micro-inserts)

How do micro-inserts work?

When the micro-inserts are in place, body tissue grows into them and blocks the fallopian tubes. It takes about three months for the tubes to be completely blocked. This prevents an egg from meeting any sperm and being fertilised.

How effective are micro-inserts?

Micro-inserts are more than 99.5 per cent effective.

Why would I want to choose micro-inserts?

The reasons for choosing micro-inserts are similar to the reasons people choose any permanent method of contraception. The special thing about micro-inserts is that you do not need a general anaesthetic, and the procedure does not involve cutting through your skin, so there will be no scars. Your fallopian tubes are not cut, clipped or cauterised either, so the procedure is a bit easier on your body and you will tend to recover more quickly than with other methods.

Are there any reasons why I could not have micro-inserts?

You cannot have micro-inserts if you have cervicitis that has not been treated. Cervicitis is inflammation of the cervix. You also cannot have micro-inserts if you have had a pelvic infection recently, or cancer of the uterus, or if your uterus is an unusual shape that makes it difficult to place them in the openings to the fallopian tubes. If there is a chance that you might be pregnant then you will have to wait until you are sure that you are not pregnant before having the procedure. You should use another effective method of contraception if you have sex during that time. You may also be asked to have some other tests done before having the procedure and a Pap test if you are due for one.

Are there any other things that could cause problems with micro-inserts?

Some medications could be a problem. Tell your doctor if you are taking any medication or have any allergies to medication, to be sure it is alright. Complications with the procedure are rare, but your doctor can tell you about anything you should know.

HOW ARE THE MICRO-INSERTS PUT IN PLACE?

The best time to have the procedure is between the seventh day after your period starts and the fourteenth day after your period starts. This is the time when the specialist will be able to see the openings to the fallopian tubes most easily, and the risk of being pregnant is reduced.

The procedure is usually done with a local anaesthetic and takes about 30 minutes. The micro-inserts are placed one after the other in each fallopian tube, using a special instrument called a hystero-scope. There is a tiny camera attached to it so that the doctor can see what to do. The hysteroscope, which is like a narrow tube, goes into the vagina then through the cervix into the uterus. It releases the micro-inserts into the openings to the fallopian tubes one at a time, where they expand to fill the first part of each tube.

WHAT CAN I EXPECT AFTER THE MICRO-INSERTS HAVE BEEN PUT IN PLACE?

When the micro-inserts are being put in place, or just after the proce-dure, you may have some cramping (like period cramps) and some bleeding. You may even feel sick for a little while, but these feelings usually don't last very long. Some women don't feel anything much at all. You will be able to go home two to three hours after the proce-dure. Any pain or discomfort in your abdomen or bleeding from your vagina should be over within three days.

During the three months it takes for the fallopian tubes to become completely blocked, you will not be able to rely on the micro-inserts for contraception. If you have sex during this time, you will need to use some other method to protect you from getting pregnant, so talk to your doctor about this before the procedure.

Three months after the procedure, you may be asked to have a special kind of X-ray to make sure the fallopian tubes are blocked. Your doctor will explain it to you. Some doctors no longer feel this test is necessary and don't do it as a routine. Once you have been told the procedure has been successful, you can stop using any other method of contraception.

Where do I get micro-inserts?

You must see your local doctor or a doctor at a Family Planning centre to get a referral to a specialist who has been trained to do the procedure. You will go to a public or private hospital to have the procedure.

What do micro-inserts cost?

The cost for two micro-inserts is about $1100, although they are available free in a few public hospitals. If you are in a medical fund you can claim the cost of micro-inserts and hospital fees, depending on your level of cover. If you are not in a fund then you need to ask the doctor about the cost. You will need to pay for the micro-inserts themselves and probably have to pay the difference between the specialist's fee and the Medicare rebate. Be sure to sort out the costs before you book in for the surgery, and to check first with your health fund if you are thinking of making a claim through them.

Frequently asked questions about micro-inserts

Q Do I have to get my partner's consent if I want to have micro-inserts?

A No, as with other methods of sterilisation, you don't need your partner's consent. It is good to talk over such a big decision together and it is best if you agree. However, in the end it is your body and your decision.

Q If I have micro-inserts, will that bring on menopause?

A No, micro-inserts have no effect on menopause. Your ovaries function as usual and you still have periods until you would normally experience menopause.

Q Will the micro-inserts affect the way I feel about sex?

A Micro-inserts have no physical effect on your body other than to block the egg from meeting a sperm and being fertilised. So they should not affect the way you feel about sex except that you may enjoy it more if you feel relieved that you will not get pregnant.

Q Can you have an operation to remove the micro-inserts so that you can get pregnant again?

A It is extremely unlikely that there is any way to reverse the blockage caused by the micro-inserts so that you could get pregnant again. You must look on having micro-inserts as absolutely permanent.

If you have any doubts about having this procedure, it is best to wait and use another method of contraception until you feel sure it is what you want. Then if your life changes in ways you had not imagined, and you regret having the micro-inserts, you will know that you had really felt it was the best decision at the time.

Things to think about if you are considering micro-inserts

» It is usually best to have micro-inserts separate from other big events in your life, especially if they are stressful. You are more likely to regret having micro-inserts if they are done when you have an abortion, or straight after you have a baby, or if you are having problems with your relationship.

» If you have micro-inserts for medical reasons, rather than because you chose to have them, you may have a lot of mixed feelings about it. You could find that talking to a counsellor or trusted friend or family member helps.

» Only choose sterilisation after thinking it over very carefully. If you already have children, you need to feel as sure as possible that no matter what happens in your life you would not want to have another child. If you have never had children, then it may be an even bigger decision to make.

» If you have micro-inserts it is even less likely that the procedure can be reversed than with other methods of sterilisation. So there is practically no chance of you ever being able to have another baby.

 HOW TO SAY THESE WORDS

cervicitis *ser-viss-eye-tiss*

Essure *ess-shore*

hysteroscope *his-ter-owe-scope*

micro-inserts *my-crow in-serts*

MALE STERILISATION (VASECTOMY)

When a man is sterilised, he has a small operation to block off the tubes that carry sperm, and then he cannot make a woman pregnant any more. The tubes that are blocked are called the vas deferens, though we usually just call them the 'vas' for short. The sterilisation procedure for men is called vasectomy, and in this session I will imagine you are a man who is interested in vasectomy and talk to you accordingly.

All the things we mentioned when we talked about tubal ligation apply to vasectomy too. If you are married or in a long-term relationship, you will probably be looking at vasectomy as a couple. The decision will affect you both, but ultimately it is your decision. You should think very carefully before choosing sterilisation because it is a permanent method of contraception. If you already have children, you need to feel as sure as possible that no matter what happens in your life, you would not want to have another child. If you have never had children, then it may be an even more difficult decision for you to make and it should not be made in a hurry.

What is a vasectomy?

When a man has a vasectomy, the tubes that carry sperm are cut and tied off or blocked off permanently (see illustration opposite).

Are there different types of vasectomy?

There are not a lot of different ways of doing a vasectomy. It can be done under general anaesthetic or under local anaesthetic if the vas are easy to feel and the man has no medical problems that might make the surgery more difficult. Some doctors make an incision on each side of the scrotum, one for each vas. Other doctors make only one incision at the midline of the scrotum and access each vas through that.

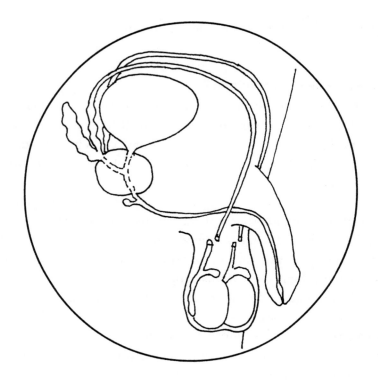

Male sterilisation (vasectomy)

How does vasectomy work?

There are two vas tubes, and each connects to one of the testes or balls on each side of the scrotum. They carry the sperm
away from the testes. Both vas feed into a single tube, called
the urethra. The urethra passes through the prostate, the bladder and then the penis.

After a vasectomy, the sperm cannot get past the blockage
made by the operation to mix with fluid called semen that normally carries the sperm from the man's body to the woman's
body when he ejaculates, or 'comes'. If no sperm enter the

woman's body, no egg can be fertilised and she cannot become pregnant.

How effective is vasectomy?

Vasectomy is very effective. It's probably one of the most effective methods, apart from not having sex. If 1000 men (remember this is 1000 not 100) used vasectomy as their method of contraception for a year, only one or two of their sexual partners would become pregnant.

It takes a while for a vasectomy to become effective. That is because there are sperm already stored on the other side of the blockage and it takes several ejaculations before they are all used up. It is very rare, but it is possible for the tubes to join up again by themselves. If this happens then a pregnancy could occur even many years after the vasectomy operation.

Why would I want to choose a vasectomy?

You may want to choose a vasectomy if you have all the children you want and you feel sure that no matter what happens, you would not want to have any more children.

You may choose vasectomy even if you have never had children and you feel absolutely convinced that you won't ever want a child, or if there is a genetic reason why you should not father any children.

If you and your partner have decided that sterilisation is the best option for you as a couple, and you have to choose between vasectomy and tubal ligation then vasectomy is often a better choice. Compared with tubal ligation, vasectomy is more effective. The procedure takes less time (either as an outpatient or in a clinic) and recovery is usually quicker. But it's important that you feel comfortable with the decision, and you are not agreeing to do it just to please your partner.

Are there any reasons why I could not have a vasectomy?

Generally, you need to talk over some issues with a doctor to find out if you can have a vasectomy. Some things that might make vasectomy more difficult, at least under a local anaesthetic, include medical problems such as diabetes and epilepsy, bleeding disorders or if you are on anticoagulant therapy, or if you have any lumps in your testes that have not yet been diagnosed.

There are some conditions that need to be treated before you can have a vasectomy. These include high blood pressure, a tendency to bleed, and any infection or dermatitis on the skin of the scrotum.

Are there any reasons why I could not have a vasectomy with a local anaesthetic?

A vasectomy may not be possible with local anaesthetic for any of these reasons:

» You have had surgery on your scrotum or it has been injured in the past. The issue here is that there may be a lot of scar tissue, which would make the vas hard to move. If the vas can't be moved easily, the procedure would be painful even with a local anaesthetic. It really would be better to have the vasectomy under general anaesthetic in hospital. The doctor will recommend the best procedure for you.

» You are very overweight. This can make it hard to feel the vas easily within the scrotum.

» You feel very nervous about having the vasectomy and really want to have it done under a general anaesthetic.

» Your scrotum has skin that is unusually thick or very tight.

» When you are examined it is found that you need to have surgery under general anaesthetic for something else, like repairing a hernia. It is usually better to have the vasectomy done at the same time.

» You have a varicose vein in the scrotum. The doctor may be concerned that you might bleed a lot during the procedure.

» You have had a lot of infections in your genital tract in the past. This can also lead to scarring, which can make the operation more difficult and painful.

WHAT HAPPENS WHEN I HAVE A VASECTOMY?

Most doctors or centres that perform vasectomies will ask you to come in to see them first to talk about the procedure before you actually make a booking to have the vasectomy. The doctor will also examine you and make sure you are suitable to have a vasectomy with a local anaesthetic if that is what is planned.

The doctor will tell you what is going to happen during the operation, and answer any questions you may have. It's important that you are clear about what vasectomy will mean for you, and what to expect. If you are in a relationship, it is good if your partner can come to this appointment as well, but it is not essential.

If you are able to have the operation and you want to go ahead with it, you will sign a consent form and make a booking for the vasectomy at the end of this visit. You will be given instructions on how to prepare for the operation before you leave.

If you are having the operation at the doctor's surgery or at a clinic, you will probably be asked to shave the pubic hair around the base of your penis and scrotum just before you go to the clinic to have the operation. If the surgery is planned under local anaesthetic, you will be at the surgery or clinic for about one to two hours altogether – this includes preparation and recovery time as well as the operation itself, which usually takes about 30 minutes. If the operation is to be done in hospital under general anaesthetic then you should expect to be in hospital most of the day.

The operation is simple and straightforward. When the operation is done under local anaesthetic, you will be given an injection into the scrotum and then into each vas. This may sting a little, but most men don't mind it too much. Some doctors give a sedative, and of course there is also the option of a general anaesthetic in hospital. When the area is numb, the doctor makes a small opening on the midline of the scrotum, carefully picks up one vas at a time, cuts them and seals the ends. Some doctors make two little openings, one for each vas, and some doctors remove a small portion of each vas before sealing the ends. Remember, the area is numb so although some men say they feel a sort of tugging feeling, it does not usually hurt. The opening in the scrotum is closed with a stitch or just with a small bandaid strip.

WHAT WILL HAPPEN AFTER THE VASECTOMY?

Most men have some bruising and discomfort for a few days after the vasectomy operation. It is important to use another method of contraception, like condoms, until the semen has been tested and no sperms are found. It takes about eight weeks for you to have enough ejaculations to remove all the sperm that are stored in front of the blockages in your vas. Eight weeks after the vasectomy, you have to take a specimen of your semen to a laboratory for testing. You need to get it there within an hour of collecting the semen. It is tested to see if there are any live sperm in it.

The doctor will explain more about this, but they will either say that everything has been successful because they didn't find any sperm in the semen, or they will ask you to come back with another specimen in a month's time. If they ask you to come back, it is usually because they have found some dead sperm and they don't want to find any at all.

If they find live sperm at the eight-week check-up, the vasectomy has not been successful and the vas has most likely rejoined. Then it is up to you to decide if you want to have a repeat operation. The doctor will discuss what has happened and will help you to sort out how you feel and what you want to do.

Where do I get a vasectomy?

Some doctors do vasectomies under local anaesthetic in their surgeries. You can also have a local anaesthetic vasectomy at some public or private hospitals, or private clinics. Some of these places also offer the option of light sedation. This is a drug given intravenously that doesn't put you completely to sleep but does make you feel very relaxed and lessens any discomfort felt during the operation. Vasectomy under general anaesthetic is done in a hospital or day surgery.

What does a vasectomy cost?

The cost of the operation varies a lot depending whether you have it done by a specialist or general practitioner, in or out of hospital or under general or local anaesthetic. Medicare will cover some of the costs and in some cases so will your private health fund if you have medical insurance. Be sure to sort out the costs you will face with the doctor who will be performing the operation before you book in for surgery, and to check first with your health fund if you are thinking of making a claim through them.

Frequently asked questions about vasectomy

Q Do I need my partner's consent to have a vasectomy?

A No. Only the person having the vasectomy needs to sign the consent form. Even if you are married, you do not need your wife's consent. Of course, it is best if you have talked it over and both of you agree that it is the best decision.

Q How long do I have to wait after my vasectomy before I can have sex?

A You should wait at least a few days, but basically you should wait until you feel comfortable. It may be a few days or a couple of weeks before you feel ready. It's up to you.

Q Will having a vasectomy affect my erections or anything about the way I have sex?

A No. Everything will function as usual. The only thing that will change is that when you 'come' there will be no sperms in the fluid you ejaculate. But you won't even be able to see or feel any difference there.

Q I have heard that you can change your mind down the track and have the vasectomy reversed so you can have more children if you want to.

A Most men, but not all men, can have an operation to join the vas again, but after this they may still not be able to father a child. We don't really know why a pregnancy doesn't happen if the vas are rejoined and sperm is found in the semen again. Sometimes it just doesn't happen. The main thing is that there is no guarantee that a reversal operation will work. In fact, you have to look at vasectomy as final. So if you have any doubts, it's best to wait and use another method of contraception until you feel sure it is what you want. Then, if your life changes unexpectedly later on, you will know that it definitely was the best decision at the time and that you didn't make it lightly.

Things to think about for men considering vasectomy

» Why do you want to have a vasectomy? Do you feel absolutely sure that you want to take this permanent step to prevent you from fathering children?

» Could it be possible that you would want another child if you have children now but they died, or if your partner died or your relationship broke up?

» How would you feel if you had a new partner who wanted to have a child with you?

» Are you or your partner worried that if you have a vasectomy, sex may not be as enjoyable?

» Do you have any doubts about having a vasectomy? If you do, it is very important to talk these over with the doctor before you decide to have the vasectomy.

» Vasectomy does not protect you from sexually transmissible infections (STIs) so you may want to use condoms as well.

HOW TO SAY THESE WORDS

anticoagulant *an-tea-co-ag-you-lant*

vasectomy *vas-eck-toe-me*

12

ABORTION

BASIC FACTS ABOUT ABORTION

If your contraception fails, or you have unprotected sex, you could become pregnant. If you are two weeks overdue for a period and there is a chance that you could be pregnant, you will need to have a pregnancy test. You can buy a urine pregnancy test kit from the chemist and do it yourself at home, or you can have it done at a local doctor's surgery, a Family Planning centre, a Women's Health Centre, a chemist, or some hospital outpatient departments. If you take a urine sample for testing, make sure that the sample is from the first time you go to the toilet in the morning and it's in a very clean jar. If you see a doctor, you may also have a blood test or a pelvic exam to check for pregnancy.

If it turns out that you are pregnant and you didn't plan to be, you may feel very confused. Many people say 'I never thought this would happen to me!' Sometimes, things seem to happen so quickly once you find out that it's hard to know what to do. It is really important to talk to someone about the choices you have. Your local doctor or someone at a Family

Planning centre will be able to help you. Look in the back of this book for numbers you can ring.

Generally, your choices are to have the baby and keep it, or have the baby and give it for adoption or foster care. Depending on where you live in Australia, and what is happening in your life, you may also choose to have an abortion.

What is an abortion?

Abortion is not a method of contraception. Contraception prevents pregnancy. Abortion is a medical procedure that terminates, or ends, a pregnancy. Sometimes, abortion is called 'termination of pregnancy'.

Are there different types of abortion?

Yes, there are spontaneous abortions and induced abortions.

A spontaneous abortion is usually called a miscarriage. It happens when the uterus contracts and pushes the foetus (the baby in the womb) out before it is fully developed and can breathe by itself. Miscarriage most often happens early in a pregnancy. A woman may not even realise she has been pregnant. She may think that she is just having a very heavy period, which is a bit later than usual. Most miscarriages happen before 12 weeks of pregnancy. We often don't know why it happens, but it is a natural process and about 15 per cent of pregnancies end this way.

With induced abortion, there are several different procedures that are used for different stages of pregnancy. The most common procedure for early-stage abortion, which is done between 6 and 12 weeks after the first day of your last period, is called suction abortion or vacuum aspiration. It is a fairly simple procedure and is very safe. The procedure for later-stage abortion takes longer and is more difficult. This means there is a greater risk.

It is also possible to take medications that cause an abortion to happen. This is more common in other countries, and is only rarely done in Australia. It can only be used in very early pregnancies, under seven weeks from the first day of your last period.

If you think you might be pregnant, find out as soon as possible so that you have plenty of time to think about what you want to do. Then if you decide to have an abortion, you will be able to have the more straightforward procedure before the end of 12 weeks.

How effective is abortion?

Although there is no guarantee that abortion is 100 per cent effective, it is almost 100 per cent effective, especially if it is done after six weeks from your last period. If you have it before then, it may not be successful because the embryo is so small it could be missed.

After a later-stage abortion, you might need to have a curette, where a different instrument is used to clear the walls of the uterus so that no tissue from the pregnancy is unknowingly left inside. Tissue from the pregnancy could cause bleeding and infection if it is not completely removed.

Why would I want to choose abortion?

There could be many reasons why you would want to have an abortion. It might not be the right time in your life to have a baby. It might be that your emotional state, or your living situation or financial circumstances, would affect the wellbeing of a child or yourself if you continued with the pregnancy.

You might want to choose abortion if you have a medical condition that would make it dangerous for you to continue with a pregnancy. You might also want to have an abortion if you know that the foetus has a severe abnormality, or if the pregnancy is a result of rape or incest.

Are there any reasons why I could not have an abortion?

Abortion is not available on request in Australia. Each state has its own laws about abortion, and you may have to meet certain requirements if you want to have one. Even in states where there are fairly broad requirements, there is usually a stage of pregnancy where the line is drawn and you cannot have an abortion after that time. In some states that time is 12 weeks and abortions are not permitted after that. Other states permit abortion up to 23 weeks as long as the other conditions are met, or even later if there is a big risk to the mother, or where the baby has a severe abnormality. If you want to find out what the law requires in your state, contact a Family Planning centre or Children by Choice. The availability of a doctor willing to perform abortions may also mean that even where the state permits abortion it can be difficult for a woman to actually have one.

What happens when I have an abortion?

For abortions up to 12 weeks of pregnancy, the procedure is usually done with a local anaesthetic in a clinic or hospital. There is less risk with a local anaesthetic and you will recover more quickly, but if you prefer a general anaesthetic, it may be possible. Some clinics have another type of anaesthetic, which is given intravenously. It is called light sedation. Sometimes it is called 'twilight sleep'. While this type of sedation does not put you completely to sleep, most women remember very little about the abortion when they wake up. You can ask about this as well when you first talk to your doctor or a counsellor about abortion.

When you go to the clinic or hospital, you may be given some medication to relax you before the procedure. The doctor performing the abortion will give you a pelvic exam and put a speculum in your vagina. A speculum is a type of instrument that can be slowly opened in your vagina to hold the vaginal walls apart so that the doctor can see your cervix easily.

If you are having a local anaesthetic then it is given into your cervix, and although some women find it a bit uncomfortable, others are not bothered by it at all. If you are having a general anaesthetic or sedation, this is usually given before the speculum is inserted into your vagina.

When the cervix is numb, the opening is slowly stretched to allow a narrow soft plastic tube to go through into the uterus. The tube is attached to a machine that uses gentle suction to remove the contents of the uterus. This all takes about 10 to 15 minutes. When the procedure is finished, you will need to rest for a while before leaving so that the doctor can be sure you are recovering as expected. If you have asked to have sedation, you may be asked to wait a little longer in the clinic until you wake up completely and you won't be allowed to drive yourself home.

After 12 weeks of pregnancy, some abortions are still done in clinics but many are done in a public or private hospital. Up to 20 weeks of pregnancy, many doctors will use a method that uses small sticks of dried seaweed, which are put into the cervix (opening of the uterus) and gradually swell up so that they slowly expand the opening. This can make some women feel crampy and nauseated but usually means that the doctor can use a slightly larger suction tube to remove the foetus from inside the uterus the following day, without too much discomfort.

Another method involves injecting hormones and saline into the uterus to make it contract. As it contracts, it eventually pushes the foetus out. It can take between 12 and 36 hours for the abortion to be completed and the contractions may feel like labour pains. After a later abortion, it may be necessary to have another procedure to make sure any tissue that may have been left in the uterus is removed.

What can I expect after the abortion?

Most women have some bleeding and period-like cramps for several days up to a couple of weeks after an abortion. Some women don't have any bleeding at all. Some women feel sick in the stomach and rather tired straight after the abortion. It is good if you can have someone with you to take you home. You should not drive, so if there is nobody to take you, plan to get a taxi. If you work, you will probably need to take the rest of the day off to recover.

Your next period will probably come between four to eight weeks afterwards. If you start on the Pill right away, your period should come when you finish all the hormone pills in the pack. You may feel very emotional for a few weeks after the abortion. Emotions can range from depression to relief and everything in between. If you feel this way, it is good to talk to someone like a close friend or a counsellor to help you through that time.

Where can I get an abortion?

You will need to talk to someone in your state to find out where you can get an abortion. Otherwise, check the telephone book in your state under 'abortion', or 'pregnancy termination services', or contact a Family Planning centre, a Community Health centre or a Women's Health Centre for a referral.

What does it cost?

The cost of abortion varies depending on the type you have

and the clinic or hospital concerned. It is best to ask about the cost when you enquire about abortions in your state.

Frequently asked questions about abortion

Q Will I be able to get pregnant again if I have an abortion?

A There should be no problem becoming pregnant again. The reason people are concerned about this is that there is a risk of infection after an abortion. If an infection travels into the fallopian tubes and is not treated quickly, scar tissue may block the tubes and prevent further pregnancies. This type of infection was much more common when abortions were done secretly by people with no medical training. If you are under the care of a doctor, you will be told about the signs of infection and, if necessary, you can be treated before any infection progresses.

Q Does my partner have to give consent for me to have an abortion?

A No, although if you are in a relationship with someone it is good to be able to talk it over and best if you agree, but ultimately it is your decision.

Things to think about if you are considering abortion

» It is very important to talk to someone such as a doctor or pregnancy counsellor about an unplanned pregnancy and the choices you have, as soon as possible.

» If you are unable to have a lawful abortion, find out all that you can about the services available to help you, whether you keep the baby or have it fostered or adopted. Never consider having an illegal abortion. An illegal abortion can be very dangerous.

» If you have an unplanned pregnancy in difficult circum-stances then you may have some regrets later on, no matter what decision you make. The important thing is to consider all your options very carefully before you decide. Then if you do have some regrets in the future, you will know that you really did what you thought was best at the time.

🐷)) HOW TO SAY THESE WORDS

curette *kew-ret*

speculum *speck-you-lim*

vaccuum *vack-youm*

aspiration *ass-per-ay-shun*

13

WHAT'S NEW?

The new methods I will tell you about in this section are not available in Australia at present, but if you are interested then you may want to ask about them over the next few years. Some of the products are already available in other countries. Each country has its own ways of testing a product to make sure the product meets with that country's regulations. So, although a contraceptive may be available overseas, it will not be approved for use in Australia without being tested here to make sure it meets our own standards.

Some new products include: contraceptive patches, combined injectables, male hormonal contraception, a combined contraceptive pill for women that does not have a break from hormone pills, and some other types of contraceptive skin implants. Let's look more closely at each of these.

THE CONTRACEPTIVE PATCH

What is the contraceptive patch?

The contraceptive patch is an adhesive patch that you wear on your skin to prevent pregnancy. It has now been approved for use in Australia, but is not being sold here at present. You can contact your doctor or a Family Planning centre to check if it is available.

How does the contraceptive patch work?

The patch contains the hormones oestrogen and progestogen, which work in your body the same way as the combined oral contraceptive pill. The hormones are released into your body from the patch, through your skin into the blood stream.

How effective is the contraceptive patch?

It is at least as effective as the combined oral contraceptive pill.

Why would I want to choose a contraceptive patch?

You may want to choose the contraceptive patch if you like the reliability of the Pill, but have trouble remembering to take it every day. The contraceptive patch will be another alternative for women who have digestive problems that prevent them from taking the Pill, or for women who don't like swallowing tablets.

Are there any reasons why I could not use a contraceptive patch?

You may not want to use the contraceptive patch if you do not want anyone to see that you are using this method. Even though you can wear the patch anywhere on your body except your breasts, you may still think that this is a problem. Some women may find that the patch does not stick to their skin very well or leaves a hard-to-remove black rim. You have to remember to replace the patch every seven days. If you cannot take the combined oral contraceptive pill for health reasons, you will not be able to use the contraceptive patch.

HOW DO I USE A CONTRACEPTIVE PATCH?

You will get a prescription from the doctor and buy the patches at the chemist. You can put the patches on yourself. Each patch lasts for a week. You use three patches in a row and then have a week's break from the hormones, just as you would with the combined oral contraceptive pill. You would expect to have some bleeding during this week when you are not using the patch. Then you start with the patches again. You can keep on with this method as long as it suits you.

COMBINED INJECTABLE CONTRACEPTION

What is combined injectable contraception?

For many years in Australia we have had progestogen-only contraceptive injections available. This type of contraception is often called DMPA, and we have already talked about this method in Chapter 5. A combined injectable contraception that contains both oestrogen and progestogen has now been developed, but is still not available in Australia.

How does the combined injectable work?

The combined injectable will act on your body in the same way as the combined oral contraceptive pill.

How effective is the combined injectable?

It is more effective than the combined oral contraceptive pill because there is no need to remember to take it every day.

Why would I want to choose combined injectable contraception?

Periods tend to become more regular after the first few months for women using a combined injectable. This is different to a progestogen-only injection, where periods are likely to be quite irregular until you stop using it. The combined injectable also reverses much more quickly than the progestogen-only injection, which means that if you wanted to, it is possible you could become pregnant a couple of months after you stop having the injections.

You have to go to the doctor every month for an injection, but for women who find that the combined hormones suit them, it can be a good choice. Researchers are looking at developing a self-injection system that should make things easier. The injection itself is relatively painless.

> **HOW DO I USE COMBINED INJECTABLE CONTRACEPTION?**
> You have the injection every thirty days, plus or minus three days.

MALE HORMONAL CONTRACEPTION

What is male hormonal contraception?

Male hormonal contraception is a method of contraception containing hormones that a man will be able to take to stop his body from producing sperm. The man will still have semen, that is, the fluid that he ejaculates, but there will not be any sperm (or only very small numbers of sperm) in it. If the man has no sperm or very small numbers of sperm in his semen and he has sex with a woman, she is very unlikely to get pregnant.

How does male hormonal contraception work?

We have known for some years that giving a man the hormone progestogen stops his body from producing both sperm and the male hormone testosterone. The progestogen can be given either as a daily pill or as an injection. But men need normal levels of testosterone to keep them healthy and to enable them to have an erection. So while the man is taking the progestogen, he is also given an implant containing enough testosterone to keep levels of this hormone normal. The implant is inserted under the skin of his abdomen and slowly releases the testosterone into his system.

How effective is male hormonal contraception?

In trials of men using this method, 80 per cent of men had no sperm in their semen and the rest had such low numbers of sperm that it would be very unlikely for their partners to fall pregnant. And there were very few side effects in men who were using this method.

At present, male hormonal contraception is only available by joining a clinical trial. Trials are being run in Australia as well as the United Kingdom and the United States. It may be a few years before male hormonal contraception is widely available.

EXTENDED-USE COMBINED ORAL CONTRACEPTIVE PILLS

A type of combined contraceptive pill that does not have a pill-free break is now available in the United States and parts of Europe. It is promoted as 'bleed-free', because you take a hormone pill every day and you don't have periods. It is a very reliable contraceptive method, but breakthrough bleeding is a common side effect when women first use the continuous pill.

OTHER CONTRACEPTIVE SKIN IMPLANTS

There are other types of progestogen-only contraceptive skin implants available in many countries throughout the world. One called Jadelle® has two rods, and another called Nor-plant® has six rods that are all implanted under the skin of the upper arm. A new type of progestogen in an implant made of silicone rubber has also been developed and is under review.

 HOW TO SAY THESE WORDS

Testosterone *tess-toss-ter-rone*

CONCLUSION

Well, we have come to the end of our sessions together. We have talked about all the methods of contraception that are available in Australia at present, and some that probably will be available in the near future, so you have plenty to think about. I know it's a lot of information, but as you read over the sessions, the methods that feel right to you will become clearer. If you have a partner, talk it over together if it's at all possible. It's good if you can agree on the method you choose.

There are many things that might influence your choice. If you feel that an unexpected pregnancy would be a serious problem for you at this time in your life, but you may want to become pregnant later on, then you need to think about using a very effective but reversible method such as the Pill or a contraceptive implant. If you have a health condition that prevents you from using hormonal methods, you may choose to look at copper IUDs or barrier methods.

If you feel that you never want to have children, or you don't want any more children, then you could include sterilisation in your options. There are other issues you might need to think about, such as the cost, how easy it is to get the method, whether you are in a sexual relationship at the moment and how comfortable you feel about using the particular method.

Now that you have a better understanding of each of the methods of contraception, you should feel more confident when you discuss your choices with a doctor or nurse. Of course there is more to know, so if you have any further questions about the different methods then contact your local doctor, a Family Planning centre, a Women's Health Centre, a Sexual Health clinic, a Community Health centre, or a natural family planning specialist. Some Family Planning centres have a telephone information line you can call. Check the 'Useful contacts' list in the back of this book or look in the telephone book for your area. You can also look on the internet, and some Family Planning centres have websites, which are also listed in the back of this book.

Oh, just a reminder – unless you are in a long-term committed relationship, no matter what method you choose, you may want to use condoms as well, because condoms help to protect you against sexually transmissible infections.

Thank you for taking the time to read this book. It is great that you care about your health and want the best for yourself. Choose well!

GLOSSARY

abortion Abortion is a medical procedure that terminates, or ends, a pregnancy. Sometimes, abortion is called 'termination of pregnancy' or TOP.

cervix The cervix is the lower part of the uterus. It is made of thick muscle that feels a bit like the tip of your nose if you touch it. The cervix sits at the far end of the vagina. At the centre of the cervix is a small opening, which is called the os. It leads to the cervical canal, which is a narrow passage that goes through to the space inside the uterus.

cystitis Cystitis is inflammation in the bladder. It causes a burning sensation when you go to the toilet and pass urine. Often, you feel that you have to go and pass urine a lot, but then when you try there's not much there at all.

ectopic pregnancy An ectopic pregnancy is a pregnancy that grows in a fallopian tube. A pregnancy in a fallopian tube has to be removed, because there is no room for it to grow and it could be very dangerous for the woman as it can cause internal bleeding.

ejaculation Ejaculation is when semen spurts out from the penis as a man has an orgasm.

embryo   An embryo is the word used for a baby that is developing in the uterus from about two weeks after fertilisation until it is about eight weeks old.

epididymis   The epididymis is a cord-like tube that stores maturing sperm that are waiting to be fed into the vas deferens. The epididymis sits along the back and to the top of each testis.

fallopian tubes   The fallopian tubes are two long, thin, hollow tubes that join onto the uterus, one on each side, and hover over the ovaries. The ends closest to the ovaries flare out like trumpets, and have tiny finger-like structures called fimbria.

Family Planning centre   Family Planning centres are special centres that provide clinics, education and information about methods of contraception. They usually offer a wide range of sexual health services as well. There is an Australian office in the ACT, called Sexual Health and Family Planning Australia, and each state has its own Family Planning centre, although the names of the centres vary. The head offices in each state are listed in the back of this book. There may be other medical clinics specifically offering family planning services in your state as well.

fertilisation   Fertilisation happens when a sperm reaches a newly released egg in one of the fallopian tubes and burrows through the egg's protective coating, so that its genes mix with those of the egg.

fertility   Fertility is the ability to start a pregnancy if you have sex without using any contraception.

hormone   A hormone is a type of chemical that is either naturally produced in a person's body or made synthetically, which regulates a particular function in the body. Sex hormones regulate the reproductive system. In hormonal contraception, synthetic hormones override the body's natural sex hormones and reduce the chances of a pregnancy.

hysterectomy   A hysterectomy is an operation to remove the uterus. It can be done through a cut in the woman's abdomen or through the vagina.

menstrual cycle   A menstrual cycle is the time between the first day of one period and the first day of the next period. During this time, under the control of hormones, a woman ovulates, and the lining of her uterus builds up and then comes away as a period (unless she has become pregnant during that cycle).

menopause   Menopause happens when a woman's hormone production changes and she stops ovulating and having periods. The average age for menopause in Australia is about 50 years.

oestrogen   Oestrogen is one of the female sex hormones that regulates the reproductive system. Natural oestrogen is made by a woman's ovaries. Synthetic oestrogen is found in the Pill and some other types of hormonal contraception.

orgasm   An orgasm happens when the muscles around the genital area in a man or a woman contract strongly again and again, and a sensation of intense pleasure and then relaxation follows.

ova   The ova are usually called eggs. One of the ova is called an 'ovum'. A human ovum is a female reproductive cell which, if it is fertilised, may grow into another human being.

ovaries The ovaries are the two glands where eggs, or ova, are produced in a woman. They sit in the woman's abdomen, one on each side of the uterus. They are joined to the uterus by strong bands of tissue that anchor them in place. The word for one of the ovaries is 'ovary'. Each ovary is oval-shaped and about the size of an olive, and contains thousands of tiny egg follicles that have the potential to produce mature eggs.

progestogen Progestogen is a synthetic hormone found in the Pill and other types of hormonal contraception. Progestogen was designed to be similar to the natural hormone progesterone, which is produced by the ovaries in a woman's body to regulate her reproductive system.

prostate gland The prostate gland is part of a man's reproductive system. It is where the sperm mix with semen, which is fluid that nourishes the sperm and carries them along and out of the man's body. The prostate is also where the part of the urethra that is connected to the bladder can be closed off, so that only semen is released when a man ejaculates. Sometimes as a man gets older, the prostate can get bigger and start to block off the flow of urine as well.

scrotum The scrotum is a loose bag of skin just behind a man's penis. It contains the two testes, or balls, that produce sperm.

semen Semen is the fluid that is ejaculated along with the sperm when a man has an orgasm. If a man has had a vasectomy, the semen no longer contains any sperm.

sexually transmissible infection A sexually transmissible infection, or STI, is an infection that is passed on through sexual contact with a person who already has the infection.

sperm   A sperm is a male reproductive cell, which can fertilise a female's ova or egg so that it grows into another human being.

testes   The testes are the glands where a man's sperm are produced. They also produce the hormone testosterone. Two testes usually sit inside the scrotum, directly behind a man's penis. The word for one of the testes is 'testis'. Each testis is egg-shaped, and about the size of a walnut. Testes are commonly called 'balls'.

urethra   The urethra is a narrow tube that carries urine from the bladder when a person goes to the toilet. In a man, the urethra also carries semen when he ejaculates. When a man is about to ejaculate, the urine is blocked from entering the urethra so that only semen is allowed to pass through.

uterus   The uterus is shaped like an upside-down pear and is normally about 6 centimetres long and 3 centimetres wide. It is made of very strong muscle that can not only stretch to accommodate a growing baby, but can also contract so strongly during childbirth that it pushes the baby out. The uterus is sometimes called 'the womb'.

vagina   The vagina is the passage that leads from a woman's vulva in between her legs to her uterus. It is usually between 6 centimetres and 10 centimetres long. When there is nothing inside it, the sides collapse onto each other so that it looks like it is closed and there is no space inside. The vaginal walls are loose and have folds. They can stretch easily too.

vas deferens   The vas deferens is usually just called 'the vas'. These are two long, narrow tubes, one vas leading away from each testis, carrying sperm to the urethra. The vas loop around the bladder and feed into the prostate gland where they join the urethra

vulva   The vulva is a word used when we talk about a woman's genital area. The vulva includes the labia, the clitoris, and the opening to the vagina.

REFERENCES

Billings, Dr Evelyn and Westmore, Ann. *The Billings Method: using the body's natural signal, of fertility to achieve or avoid pregnancy*, revised edn. Melbourne: Anne O'Donovan Pty Ltd, 2000.

Contraception: an Australian clinical practice handbook, 2nd edn, Sydney: Sexual Health & Family Planning Australia, 2008.

Guillebaud, John. *Contraception: Your Questions Answered*, Edinburgh: Harcourt Publishers Limited, 1999.

Guillebaud, John. *The Pill and other forms of hormonal contraception*, 5th edn, New York: Oxford University Press, 1998.

Szarewski, A. Guillebaud, J. *Contraception: a user's guide*, 3rd edn, New York: Oxford University Press, 2000.

The 2001 Guidelines for Clinical Practice, Sydney: FPA Health, 2001.

USEFUL CONTACTS

**SHFPA
(SEXUAL HEALTH AND FAMILY PLANNING
AUSTRALIA)**

GPO Box 2138
Canberra ACT 2601
Ph: (02) 6230 5255
Website: www.shfpa.org.au

ACT

SHFPACT
Sexual Health & Family Planning ACT
Suite 4, Level 1
28 University Avenue
(GPO Box 1317)
Canberra ACT 2601
Ph: (02) 6247 3077
Website: www.shfpact.org.au

New South Wales

Family Planning NSW

328-336 Liverpool Rd
Ashfield NSW 2131
PH: (02) 8752 4300
Healthline: 1300 65 88 86
Website: www.fpnsw.org.au

Northern Territory
FPWNT
Family Planning Welfare Association of NT
Head Office & Darwin Clinic
Unit 2 The Clock Tower
Coconut Grove NT 0810
Ph - Clinic: (08) 8948 0144
Ph - Admin & Education: (08) 8948 0326
Website: www.fpwnt.com.au

Queensland
Family Planning Queensland (FPQ)
100 Alfred St
(PO Box 215)
Fortitude Valley QLD 4066
Ph - Clinic: (07) 3250 0200
Ph - Education: (07) 3250 0240
Website: www.fpq.com.au

South Australia
SHine SA (Sexual Health information networking and
education)
64c Woodville Road
Woodville SA 5011
Ph: (08) 8300 5300
1300 883 793

1800 188 171
Website: www.shinesa.org.au

Tasmania
Family Planning Tasmania
2 Midwood St
Newtown TAS 7002
(PO Box 77 North Hobart TAS 7002)
Ph - Clinic: (03) 6228 5244
Ph - Admin: (03) 6228 5422
Website: www.fpt.asn.au

Western Australia
FPWA (formerly Family Planning Western Australia)
70 Roe St
Northbridge WA 6003
 (PO Box 141 Northbridge WA 6865)
Ph: (08) 9227 6177
Infoline (08) 9227 6178
1800 198 205
Website: www.fpwa.org.au

Victoria
Family Planning Victoria
901 Whitehorse Road
(PO Box 1377)
Boxhill VIC 3128
Ph - Admin: (03) 9257 0100
Website: www.fpv.org.au

Look in the White Pages of your telephone book or online for other services, for example:

» contraception *see* Family Planning
» natural family planning *see* natural family planning *or* Billings family planning
» Sexual Health clinics *see* Sexual Health clinics
» Community Health centres *see* Community Health centres
» Women's Health Centres *see* Women's Health Centres
» abortions *see* abortion services
» counselling about relationships *see* Relationships Australia